Who is the Pale Pony? Listen . . .
My name is Chronic Illness.
You can no longer go where you want to go —
when you choose —
at the speed you pick.
That's true because I will give you weakness
instead of strength.
Excitement and pride?
Never again will you have them like before!
I plan only confinement
and disability for you.
And I will be your constant companion.

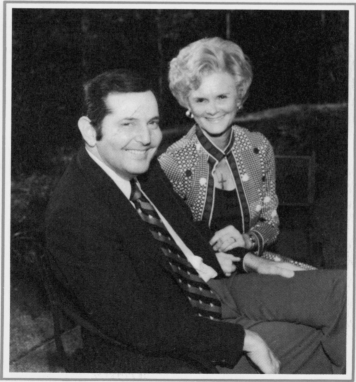

Photo by William C. Connell, Jr. of Oxford, Mississippi.

Ronald and Myra Sue Pruet

RUN FROM THE PALE PONY

RUN FROM THE PALE PONY
Coping with Chronic Illness

Ronald B. and Myra Sue Pruet

BAKER BOOK HOUSE
Grand Rapids, Michigan

Copyright 1976 by
Baker Book House Company

ISBN: 0-8010-6994-7

Printed in the United States of America

First printing, May 1976
Second printing, November 1976

With love, gratitude, respect, and honor,
Myra Sue and I dedicate this story to
my parents,
C. B. and Aileen Pruet

Contents

Foreword

About thirty years ago one of my joys as a boy was to ride a white horse named Prince. That proud, spirited stallion carried me where I wanted to go—whenever I bid him to— at the pace which I chose.

I don't have to explain to horsemen the feeling of strength, even authority, which comes from controlling such a powerful animal. Nor need I expand on the excitement I felt when I galloped Prince at full speed, or about the quiet pride that came when I twisted him through the corkscrew turns of a rodeo exercise. After all, he was mine, and I had trained him.

Those experiences are part of my heritage.

My cherished white horse was gone and seldom remembered about fifteen years later. It was then I encountered a completely different kind of steed.

When I first became aware of the specter, its shape was too dim to discern. I knew only that I had never seen anything like it before. Too, I knew that I had not sought any such creature. Yet "something" different was with me wherever I went—and the shadow would not go away.

I told myself, "Really now! You are much too busy to bother with something that seems determined to disturb you. Get rid of it!"

And I tried to will it away.

No matter what I did though, the specter followed my every move. Furthermore, the harder I tried to lose it, the clearer the creature's form became to me.

My uneasiness changed into anxiety when I realized that this unwanted shadow had a will of its own. The chill of fear came when I understood that it had no intention to leave me alone.

Without further warning it began to communicate openly with me one day. In a harsh voice which was almost rigid with animosity it spat out,

You can no longer go where you want to go—when you choose—at the speed you pick.
That's true because I will give you weakness instead of strength.
Excitement and pride? Never again will you have them like before! I plan only confinement and disability for you!!
And I will be your constant companion.
My name is Chronic Illness!!!

At the time I heard it speak, I shrank back from actually seeing it face to face. It spoke harshly of miseries which were inverse to joys with my white horse named Health, and the bitter irony was reflected in the form of the malicious creature. Chronic Illness took the shape of a stunted, misshapen pony.

Its shaggy coat was pale in color, streaked with ages-old accumulations of dark despair. But unquestionably the most frightening feature of the animal was its overwhelming, glare-eyed stare which held me helpless. The pony's wild eyes darted restlessly from side to side; yet strangely they were unblinking. I had never seen an expression in the eyes of man or beast which was so malevolent as when it spewed out what it intended for me.

This book is written first of all for those people who have met the Pale Pony face to face. There are ever so many causes of the confrontation, including serious physical or mental illness, accident, and war injury. But the results are quite similar.

The Pale Pony, Chronic Illness, speaks in the same vicious language to us all.

What's more, the Pale Pony does not overlook those people who are close to the ones he selects. Often the loved ones, the indirect victims, suffer fully as much as those with chronic illness, though of course not in the same manner. To those people too this book is addressed.

A third target group includes the professionals who minister daily to the ones who are directly and indirectly affected by chronic illness. Their tasks may vary from medically treating physical and mental illness to offering spiritual advice and consolation. Their experience may be ever so broad, but that ministry might be made a tiny bit more effective by considering this fresh view from one who has met the Pale Pony, reflected upon common struggles, and written it down.

I don't pretend great medical or religious knowledge; nor would I suggest a heretofore secret cure for what ails you, yours, or those you visit. What we do share in *Run from the Pale Pony*, however, are verbal pictures of very real experiences of family members responding to a serious illness.

Furthermore, I don't claim that we are a unique family— far from it. The number of people who are in a similar situation is quite large, and other answers to chronic illness may be more heroic or even superior to ours. I will say this though: We are meeting daily problems now in such a way that all members of our family are happy, productive, and secure.

Before I go any further, you must understand that the purpose of this book is to offer *hope,* not a prediction of defeat at the hands of the Pale Pony. Even more, I suggest that if we can't tame the Pony, both yours and mine, we will at least disrupt his plan for us.

Part One of the book is the section in which I tell about experiences and emotions which I had when I met my Pale Pony. I whisk you from the West Texas plains through a hospital in Abilene, Texas, into the Mayo Clinic in Rochester, Minnesota, and then all the way through a complete turnaround in my life direction.

Incidentally, this is your written guarantee that those hospital stays that I lead you through will be absolutely painless and will not harm you in any way. Surprisingly, we even find quite a bit of humor in one hospital we visit.

In Part Two I propose a way to compare "where you are," so to speak, to "where you want to be" in the course of any long-term affliction. Of course I realize that in the end nearly all of us want to be free of the Pale Pony. Until that happens though, this new system will help you judge just "where you are." Maybe then you can improve your position.

After examining that new way to measure chronic illness, we explore eight different "wiggles," that is, ways that I have used in trying to shake my uninvited guest. I would be willing to wager that you have tried most of them yourself if you're acquainted with the Pony.

Part Two ends with what could be called my philosophy of chronic illness. Instead of naming it so grandly, however, I'd rather say that in Part Two I discuss the five action-commitments which have helped me most during these last fourteen years with the Pale Pony.

Part Three discloses my wife's reactions to my long affliction. My mate, Myra Sue, supplies vivid descriptions of the emotions and trials of one who is vitally—even though indirectly—affected by chronic illness. She begins by telling of family foundations and experiences.

Next she shares her inner feelings and delayed responses to my chronic illness. Her emotions were so deep that she was snared by her own Pale Pony. She ends by telling of thoughts that she carries now as well as thoughts that lift her in coping with the Pale Pony.

The Epilog not only suggests how the Pale Pony began but also points to the time it was conquered. You don't have to accept its message, but I challenge you to think about it.

PART ONE

Meeting the Pale Pony

1

Puzzle Without a Solution

Something was wrong! Have you ever been to a point where questioning simply led to more questions—with no answers? That's where I was for far too long: I had lived in a scrambled mystery. Solutions were not apparent to anyone in Midland, Texas, my home in the Land of the High Sky since 1957. As a matter of fact, the problem itself was not obvious even to friends, business associates, or medical experts because there were no apparent outward signs. Nevertheless, the unanswered questions had become an increasingly heavy load to carry for Myra Sue and me during the last two years.

The last half of 1962 and the first half of 1963 were times when my wife and I searched every corner and crevice for an answer to the question, "What is physically wrong with Ronald Pruet?" Call it my "big wondering" that had grown to a point past pleading and praying to a level of demanding at least a plausible diagnosis of the set of problems.

That demand for an answer is what led me to drive eastward with my family on that hot summer day in early June 1963. As we sped along the straight Texas highway, I tried to shut out the familiar squeals of three small boys squabbling in the back of the Pontiac station wagon. Without looking back, I could sense the actions of Ron, aged 10, whose quiet mission seemed to be to lead Rick, master brother-buster at age 7, to torment Brent, age 4, whose current approach to every problem was a wail. Myra Sue, light of my life since we went together in high school, endured—seemingly lost in thought.

A welcome distraction for me in that stretch of West Texas was anticipating, identifying, and then admiring the oil well pumping units and the bright silver tank batteries scattered on each side of the highway. My education at Texas Tech in petroleum engineering and then activities as a consultant in and near the oil business for the last fourteen years had instilled a love for oil activity which was basic to my nature. Too, I had been close to the oil business long enough not to reflect—very often—what might have been if only. . . .

The 150-mile drive between Midland and Abilene passed quickly. The countryside had changed slowly from the stark plains further west to gently rolling hills, dotted with thin mesquite trees sporting their thin lace-like leaves colored bright yellow-green. Customarily, the grass was late because of sparse spring rains. Coming into town, I was still hesitant about keeping the appointment I had made earlier in the week with Dr. Azle. I pictured instead the bright blue water at Lake Leon just outside of Ranger. How much more delightful it would be for all of us to go to the cabin, unload our troubles, and dash to swim or ski! Thinking again, however, I was reminded that my troubles were not the kind that could be unloaded like a suitcase.

Decision reluctantly made, I dropped Myra Sue and the kids at her folk's house in Abilene and then drove to the doctor's office. My internal-medicine specialist there was not necessarily more knowledgeable than the Midland doctors that I had consulted; but, somehow, he inspired hope. Furthermore, when I finished talking to him that morning, he persuaded me to go one more step—enter the hospital for a complete physical. Evidently he was a master salesman. He had already checked me out in some depth about eight months earlier, but the results were inconclusive. That time he had sprung an alarming disease on me, a disease that I had heard just enough about to know that it should be avoided. One simple test, however, caused him to say that at least *that* ailment was not my trouble. The questions were still unanswered.

I left to Myra Sue the problem of properly distributing the boys among willing grandparents and assorted relatives. This reciprocal charity was necessary because no single relative was able (or willing) to handle all three boys at once for periods longer than two consecutive meals. In order to keep my hospital appointment on Sunday, the following day, we made the rounds to grandmom in Abilene and mama in Ranger. We promised each son and relative that the visit would be short because I was going in only for a check-up. Surely, we said, we will collect our brood in less than a week.

I don't know all of the reasons for that quiet feeling of personal assurance I had as we drove to the hospital on that June Sunday. The feeling was the same that one feels after he successfully completes a major problem. Perhaps in this case the confidence partially came from being in "home country," sixty miles from Ranger, that small Texas town where both Myra Sue and I were born some thirty-four years ago. I glanced at her as she rode beside me. Perhaps my confidence came from knowing I could count on my wife's presence and prayers. Maybe that imposing Baptist hospital building itself affirmed that a sound decision had been made, and that all would be well. Deep down too, there must have been hope, even faith, that God would guide because of active "Baptist support" I had given in every city where I had lived. He and I weren't strangers. Finally, like all who think themselves vigorous and self-sufficient, I believed that all physical problems in our modern age for an up to now healthy young man could be easily corrected once they were properly diagnosed. Put it all together—I was personally convinced that nothing was wrong that wouldn't be put right in this hospital in short order.

Bolstered by all those real and imagined supports as we drove up to Hendricks Memorial Hospital in Abilene, I parked the car, got out, and then, after pausing to admire the new fountain outside, quickly climbed the stairs leading inside. With an almost jaunty air, I carried a bag containing nothing more than one set of new pajamas and assorted toiletry articles. As I remember that time now, I am sure that there was a great deal of bravado in my manner as I strode to the registration desk and confirmed the arrangements made the day before. Not uncommonly, Myra Sue was talking to some acquaintance she ran across in the lobby, but she quickly followed as I went to my room on the sixth floor. Sailing smoothly on a cushion of confidence, I could see no reason to be apprehensive about a simple physical examination.

I sat on the side of the bed in my room in the "old wing" of Hendricks. The tan walls seemed familiar, perhaps because tan is the color that West Texans are exposed to daily. I remember thinking, "What a strange place to spend such a beautiful Sunday afternoon." Myra Sue sat easily in the single chair in the room, chattering about the children and then jumping abruptly to an unrelated subject. I knew that she was somehow both relieved and worried, and that the conversation was designed to reassure us both.

I was calm. After all, I mentally confirmed, I had never been admitted as a patient to any hospital in any town or city where I had lived. I had never suffered even a broken bone in spite of an active childhood and adolescence. Born and raised in the former oil boom town of Ranger, Texas, I was even a starting tackle in 1944 and 1945 for the Ranger High football team—still no hospital stay. In addition, I was active but not as proficient in tennis, track, and basketball. The most serious accident of my sporting career was a scraped nose, which was faithfully recorded in a football photograph in the high school annual. Up to now, my exposures to hospitals included only two trips in Ranger for the births of two sons and once in Midland for yet another son. There had been no complications to sons, mother, or father as a result of earlier introductions to hospital confinement. No reasons for pessimism because of past experience.

The friendly nurse brought the evening meal soon after Myra Sue left to buy a sandwich at a nearby drug store. I am quick to confirm after my evening meal that meat loaf in a hospital is unimpressive. By the time Myra Sue came back the nurses' aide had picked up the tray, and a second nurse came by to take an evening temperature. I remember thinking, "But I am not sick that way, and I would have preferred going out to eat; though I must admit I am a little tired." We found in a breezy conversation with the new nurse first that I had an uncle in a room just down the hall, and second, that she recognized that I had the same last name as an Abilene doctor. (That wasn't surprising since he is my cousin.)

Very quickly, it seemed, 9:00 P.M. came, and visiting hours were over. After reading an uninteresting magazine article, tossing quite a bit, and doing all those trivial things that one can do alone in the hospital, I decided that sleep must be summoned. Instead of sleep, however, I seemed to call up the flood of unknowns, who proceeded promptly to batter the bridge of confidence which I had just crossed. Doubt, spokesman for the "unanswered questions," led off by reviewing my recent symptoms and medical history. Soon Doubt and Confidence, each by then a separate entity in thought, carried on a conversation both with and within me which went something like this:

Doubt, that power of darkness, pointed out, You've been to four doctors in the last two years, and not one could tell you what's the matter. All I can see for your efforts is that you are getting worse—not better.

Confidence answered with feeling: So what? All you need is a physical examination that punches all the right buttons. A good doctor can map out a way to get rid of any symptom that a man in his early thirties can dream up.

Doubt: But what about that numbness in your right hand that has been there for the last two years. Don't forget that the tingling has grown in the last month from the ring and little fingers to include the whole palm of your hand.

Too you can't overlook the fact that just this last week
your right foot has the same tingling.

Confidence: So it's growing a little. That doesn't mean that it
won't go away just as quickly as it came. You must recognize too that there is absolutely no pain with that tingling
or numbness. If it doesn't hurt, it can't be all that bad!
Calm down—it will all clear up.

Doubt: Think about that tightness around your stomach. You
know very well how often lately that you tried to loosen
your belt to correct the feeling—only to find that your
belt was not tight at all. I don't mind telling you that you
got a silly expression on your face every time that happened.

Confidence: Tightness around your stomach is because of tension—plain and simple. After you get those leases signed,
it will be all right—you'll see. Say now, don't you remember way back in 1950 when you were working for
Gulf in Illinois? Your stomach was upset all of the time
because of tension. It was diagnosed as gastritis by a
St. Louis doctor, and then the trouble went away when
you took a few pills. After you relax, maybe even take
a vacation, this tightness will do the same thing as before—
go away.

Doubt: Myra Sue, the one who knows you better than anyone
else, has told you over and over that you are more tired
and irritable this year with only one job that you were
three years ago when you were handling four jobs at once—
trying to sell real estate, selling coin-op dry cleaners, op-
erating a laundromat, and turning oil deals. She says that
you come home now, seem normal as you first relax, and
then what looks like a veil comes over your eyes. She's
on record as predicting a nervous breakdown for you soon,
if you are not already into the scene.

Confidence: I don't even know what she is thinking about when
she talks like that! Veils—pooey! It doesn't seem too
much to ask of a wife that she keep the kids from yelling
and fighting when you come home from work! You may

not understand some of the problems that we may or may not have, but this much I know—you are *not* having a nervous breakdown!

Doubt: But what about this doctor of yours that has you on this wild-goose chase? Didn't he frighten you with an ailment that you had hardly heard of last October and then after one test tell you that you didn't have that illness after all? Sounds to me like he doesn't really know what he is talking about. Maybe he is just trying to earn a fat medical fee!

Confidence: Ah ha! Didn't he say that he was going to bring in another specialist, a neurologist, in your case? As a matter of fact, you already know that some of those tests that begin tomorrow are prescribed by the neurologist. Now we are getting somewhere! And don't forget too that your doctor cousin here is also an internal-medicine specialist. He will surely watch over the whole thing if you ask him to. Relax and go to sleep. A couple of days' testing will open the way to all the answers you want. Besides there's no one here now that you have to act healthy for; admit that you are tired, and go to sleep.

Doubt: But let me point this out. . . .

Back and forth it went all Sunday night, even after sleep came. My impression the next morning was that "Doubt" was persistent and more persuasive as the argument progressed.

2

Weakness and Strength

"Turn over on your side. Tuck your knees in as close to your chest as you can. Now relax."

These simple instructions came from Dr. Regenio, my neurologist, after he had popped into my room early Monday morning and had an attendant wheel me up to "surgery." As I lay in that bright white room, the first two special orders were easy, but the third was impossible. No sane person could relax after catching a glimpse of what the attending nurse was handing to the peppy little doctor—the most awesome hypodermic syringe that any patient could imagine. That silver syringe must have been well over sixteen inches long, though truth leads me to admit uncertainty about its exact length. This is because I saw the instrument only once. I was "careful" to avoid that sighting mistake in any of the four spinal taps which I have had since that fearsome first one. "Careful" is a rank understatement. I was scared spitless!

Actually a spinal tap is only a sampling of the fluid from the spinal column, searching for abnormalities in the liquid that surrounds that important protected sheath of nerves. Though I hate to admit it, the tap itself, even with the awe-inspiring syringe, was uncomfortable but not painful. It took only a few seconds. A simple but helpful truth dawned on me later: the *anticipation* of pain was far more unpleasant than

the actual experience. Unfortunately, that fact was easy for
me to believe only *after,* instead of before or during, the trying
experience.

Later that same day an intern (a graduate but apprentice
doctor) carrying a note pad, a pen, and wearing a forced smile
came to Room 609. His instructed bedside manner was much
in evidence.

"Mr. Pruet?" he questioned, affirming first that patient
matched the room number, "your doctors asked me to prepare
your complete medical history. I know that you have already
told them some of it more than once, and, of course, [chuckle]
you are going through part of it now. What I am asking is
that you tell me about every medical symptom that you ever
had, going back as far as you can remember. Now, first of all,
have you ever . . . ?"

Then followed the long list of questions which, true to his
prediction, I had already answered at least twice. Dragging
at first, I reluctantly got into the spirit of "remember when."
Give the young intern credit though, because he did help me
expand on two earlier incidents. I couldn't imagine then why
they would seem significant to the doctors in charge.

The first obscure happening came as far back as 1954, nearly
ten years earlier. The mother of a friend of mine was seriously
ill in Ranger, the town where I lived then. She needed blood
transfusions to survive, and her problems were even more criti-
cal because her blood type was relatively rare. Since my blood
type matched hers, I joined the donors' list and gave a pint
of blood, a routine act which I had done earlier several times.
For a number of days after this transfusion, however, unlike
earlier experience, there was a consistent tingling—no pain—
in my right leg. It was no big problem, but I mentioned it to
a physician friend of mine.

Adopting the "avoidance approach," Dr. Harris advised
"Don't give any more transfusions."

I didn't, and the tingling went away. Another triumph for
medical science!

The second bland incident happened around the spring of

1961, two years earlier. Remember my claiming to be a non-proficient tennis player? About that time period I either played tennis or went 200 miles to water ski during any of the rare breaks in business activity. One afternoon I was enjoying a spirited tennis match with a business associate of mine in Midland, Texas. We had a pretty fair game going, volleying back and forth. All of a sudden, one of his shots was by me without my seeing it. With all due respect, he was not that good. Then followed a couple of serves by my opponent with the same results; I could not follow the path of the ball after it left his racquet.

"L.D.," I shouted, "let's shut it down. I don't have any trouble seeing anything else, but for some reason I can't follow your serves after you hit them. Must be something wrong."

L. D. was a little upset at quitting when things were going so well, but he knew I was not throwing the game since he usually won anyway. Another day's competition would be more challenging.

Dr. Kinkaid, the opthalmologist who examined my eyes a few days later, told me, "Your trouble is caused by a small lesion in the retina of your right eye. That 'lesion' is simply a torn place, cause unknown. It could be serious if it gets larger. Let's watch it, but it will probably clear up before long."

We non-physicians can recognize that Dr. Kinkaid used the "wait a while" approach, closely akin to Dr. Harris's "avoidance approach." In this case too the doctor was right. It went away, and to this day—thank You, Lord—that lesion is the only trouble which I have had with my vision other than normal aging.

All of this conversation was faithfully recorded in my medical history. Thinking back to that time, as an aside, there is one thing I am curious about: the legibility of the records written hurriedly by interns and physicians. Although I have never seen a detailed medical record of any patient, it is hard to believe that doctors can always in later years interpret what they wrote about what they thought they heard us say.

All of the various tests that are routine to any complete

physical were quickly added to my non-routine spinal tap, supplementing the medical history as completely as possible. The stage was set for two significant things which happened during the first week after I was admitted to Hendricks Memorial. First of all, the long sought diagnosis came early. Second, a completely unsuspected physical change developed.

The morning of the third day, both Dr. Azle and Dr. Regenio came to Room 609. Myra Sue had arrived early and was relaxing in "her" chair.

Dr. Azle began in a soft, unemotional voice, "Well, Mr. Pruet, we think we have it pinned down. I have a number of patients with the same illness. We had to eliminate all of the other possibilities before deciding. But after looking at the complete picture, we agree that what's left is what you have. Some of your symptoms are a little different from my other patients, but you have many of the same complaints. Now rest easy—all my patients with that disease are doing well."

Then he began to make what may be called "the doctor's exit" from the hospital room, a quick change maneuver that means he's vanished before your very eyes, well before you can tell him that you lost your left leg last night.

Calling him back, I anxiously questioned, "But, doctor, what *is* the disease?"

"Oh, I thought I told you. You have multiple sclerosis."

"But—but, Doctor Azle," I said after a moment of stunned silence, "that's what you told me last fall that I *didn't* have!"

"Mr. Pruet, I wasn't sure then. We've run more tests this time. Enough to be sure now."

Dr. Regenio nodded his agreement, and then both doctors left quickly for more hopeful patients. Neither physician volunteered any information about the disease. Perhaps that's one reason that I have no recollection about my specific reaction to the bad news. Myra Sue tells me that I "took it well."

Parenthetically, I have still learned relatively little during the last twelve years about MS (short for multiple sclerosis). Nevertheless my required personal "research" into the mysterious disease has generated the following sparse facts: The disease which

I have affects the nervous system in general, the spinal column nerves in particular. The varied effects on the approximately 100,000 cases in the United States (a total which is always increasing) range across how we see, feel, think, walk, talk, taste, and more. There is no common denominator; that is, one effect does not necessarily lead to another; nor must each patient be afflicted to the same degree at any time.

The average age of each victim, most of whom are women living in northern latitudes, is thirty, the prime of life. The cause of MS is completely unknown. Furthermore, there is no commonly accepted treatment of its symptoms; nor, of course, is there a cure. About the only agreement about the course of the illness is that its symptoms come and go (jargonese for the medical terms *exacerbation* and *remission*). Oh, yes, doctors agree (and they back it with statistics) that some die early, say within a few months; and some live a long time (I know one lady who has had MS for fifty-two years).

How's that for a winner? I traded a puzzle without a solution for a disease without a cure.

Enough of that! No more disease education, I promise you. This book is *not* written to discuss the miscellaneous problems of MS patients; nor of those with any other specific disease, for that matter.

Instead, I feel led to share certain facts and reactions which have helped me adjust to a severe interruption in my life plan and style. Go a step further; I humbly believe that certain of these facts and responses amount to revelation.

Don't get me wrong! I *know* that there have been many who have suffered from illness more severely than I. I *know* that what applies to one individual does not necessarily apply to all. I *know* there have been many who have adjusted better than I. Believe me; I do not count myself unique. Even so, I guess I'm at least not "average."

There is, after all, nothing "average" about being told that you have one of those illnesses that has its own national society. Furthermore, two years is not the *average* time necessary to learn the name of a "mystery guest" that has taken up residence with you. In addition, I have responded to MS in several ways that might strangely be called both common and also unusual.

Say . . . I know what I want to do now.

You look like a pleasant companion. Will you join me in a very "un-average" journey? What I propose is that you come with me through the experience I had after I was "introduced to illness" in Abilene. I promise it won't hurt you no matter where we go. Also, I don't think you will be bored.

In return, I ask you to consider a few of my thoughts that apply to all long-term illnesses or accidents. Some of the things we will share just might be helpful to you or someone else whose life direction has been changed unexpectedly.

All right, all right—you get to ask questions or disagree when you want to. I don't claim to have taken every turn correctly on this journey; nor were all the decisions mine alone. Up to now though, there's light ahead instead of darkness.

Now back to the "week that was." Or—Let's start our trip!

The second happening of that eventful week came progressively in the three days after I learned the name for what was wrong. The radical physical change came so suddenly that it seemed that MS had answered my question, "What can it do?" Within one week after I came to the hospital, I was *unable to walk.* I would tell you more about the change from "briskly carrying a suitcase into the room" to "flat on my back" if I could; but, frankly it's still a mystery to me. I can only testify that by the end of the week it was so far from my bed to the bathroom in the same room that I had to have a hospital attendant help me.

As best I can learn, the general medical explanation goes like this: MS interrupts the nerve signal from the brain that tells a muscle or muscles to move in such and such a way. Since the muscle is unable to get the signal, it cannot move and thus becomes weaker and weaker from disuse. Those nerve signals can't be seen, but "weaker and weaker" was all too easy to demonstrate. Daily my doctors would ask me to stiffen my legs and then hold both above the bed. Even on the best days my right leg (one side is always weaker) would droop slowly in a few seconds, no matter how hard I tried to hold it up. On the worst days I could lift neither leg. Another simple test would be for me to wiggle each big toe—with the left usually "could do," with the right usually "no way." It was very hard to reconcile that reluctantly demonstrated weakness with the fact that only a couple of weeks earlier I had no trouble playing two or three consecutive sets of tennis.

Accompanying this transition from "go" to "can't go" was a rapid increase in the amount and severity of the tingling numbness. My right leg, beginning with my foot and moving to the calf of my leg, became numb. Of course, the "belt" across my stomach along with all the other introductory symptoms persisted. Tests to measure this effect were varied, and like the symptom, painless. One doctor used a vibrating tuning fork to test for feeling when he touched it to different affected areas. Another would often follow later with a pin and a feather, alternating and hiding each to see if I could distinguish between the two. Another challenging test, one which I tried not to flunk, was to identify a coin—nickel, penny, or quarter—when it was slipped into my palm. I was tempted to sneak a look before guessing, but finally decided that "winning" was not the point in this case.

Describing my feelings about this unexpected change in "go power" is difficult. My impression now is that I was so confident that the crippling effect would be temporary and easily corrected that I did not consider reacting with dismay. Looking back at that feeling now makes me realize that it was completely illogical to be so calm and confident. After all, I couldn't walk from "here" to "there"; yet I needed to return quickly to managing the two-year-old equipment leasing company which I had helped organize. Furthermore, though now I had a name for my troubles, I knew nothing about the disease. For overcoming those very powerful negative facts, there must have been several strong causes for my confidence.

One cause—and it's big enough to do it alone—was my rekindling of the power of individual prayer in that bedside battlefield. Of course a hospital stay is like a stand in battle! My early religious training, as well as practice as an active church worker, provided the base for an intensified—though sporadic and pleading—prayer program. In addition, I read familiar passages in the Bible. I respectfully listened to the hospital chaplain and then prayed with him. I believed then, as I do now, that neglecting the power of prayer in hospital conflict is like trying to fly with one wing! However, I cannot truthfully say that my specific prayers then were answered. I asked for complete recovery—a request yet to be granted.

Another cause, I learned later, may be tied to multiple sclerosis itself. A severe attack such as I was in then is sometimes accompanied by a feeling of euphoria, that is, a feeling of extreme happiness and well-being. Perhaps because my confidence was illogical, the doctors were right in saying it was euphoria rather than confidence. Even so, I can recall no giddy "high"; nor was I under any kind of medication that could produce one. I honestly believe that I thought in normal patterns. Still, that illogical assurance was there, and I am a logical man.

Yet another possible cause was prayer from others, usually identified in religious literature as "intercessory prayer." During that crisis period Myra Sue spent long periods in prayer and meditation, separate from the times we were together. By the end of the week, relatives and friends who lived in and near Abilene had joined in prayers of support. I have no doubt that this form of love lifted me. Yet how do you measure how much God listens to a devout relative when she comes to Him in your behalf? The answer is one short word: impossible.

Time in the hospital stretched well beyond the projected "couple of days" for a check-up. Treatment by intravenous injection (commonly known as I-V's) began, which seemed to dampen the crippling effects. Improvement to some degree came in a couple of weeks. Medication was changed, and a routine of physical therapy prescribed. Instead of improvement, the wavering, favorable changes were reversed. The therapy program included hot whirlpool baths and exercises, procedures probably very beneficial for football injuries but which com-

pletely sapped all the energy in this MS patient. By the end
of one month in the hospital I was back to where I was at the
end of one week—nowhere.

Lonesome? Depressing? Defeating? Yes, and, surprisingly,
no. Yes, for obvious reasons such as no kids allowed for hospital visits, no passes for the real world, none of the outdoor
pleasures normal for summer, uncertainties about my business,
and on and on. No, for two main reasons. The first cause was
the very reassuring friendship and love shown by family and
friends, a consistently powerful lift. The second reason was an
attitude which Myra Sue and I encouraged during the whole
hospital period. That particular outlook is usually rare to a
hospital room but is always present in a well-balanced person,
no matter what his state of health.

This second reason was simply a strong sense of humor, the
ability to laugh at both outside events and myself. I can think
of several examples which, from one point of view, could be
considered as either annoying or an outrageous imposition. From
the point of view with "sense of humor" in control, however,
these same examples were considered either so ridiculous or
amusing that they became outrageously funny to me.

The first came early in my hospital stay—soon enough that
my family (other than Myra Sue) expected me home mo-
mentarily, but before they had learned that I could not walk.
On the first day of the second week, dad called me early in the
morning, slightly before my wife's customary time of arrival
from her folk's house around 8:00 A.M. He was calling for
help in caring for Brent, our four-year-old. Somehow the children had been shuffled in the preceding weekend, resulting in
the precarious combination of brother-buster Rick and the
easily ruffled, ear-infection-prone Brent together at Mother and
Dad Pruet's home in Ranger. Not stressing my downhill development to dad, I tried to soothe the Ranger home front by
promising better advice a little later from Myra Sue if he
and mama couldn't handle my youngest.

After hanging up the phone, I decided to go to the bathroom
by myself, ignoring the warnings of my wife who had just

walked into the room. After all, I had been doing that little
chore alone for well over thirty years. 99.9 percent of the
time I am right (I try to convince myself), but this *one* time
Myra Sue called the shot on the money. I couldn't get back
to the bed from the bathroom without help. Leaning upon her,
I lurched to the bed which she had edged closer to the door,
and then sprawled across it. About the same time, the telephone
rang. It was dad again. He urgently explained in detail that
Brent was unmanageable, had refused to take his bath, and
would not eat his scrambled eggs. He was mollified when Myra
Sue suggested that Brent was probably sick and needed to
be taken to the doctor. So dad stopped well short of saying
what he must have thought—that we should pack up quickly
to reclaim the kids.

After hanging up the second phone call from the distraught
granddad, one of us glanced at my awkward stance on the
askew bed and then made some sort of remark about the "des-
perate situation" in Ranger. The remark inexplicably tickled
both our funnybones. When a nurse happened by, she found
both of us in uproarious laughter. She paused a moment and
then left for my doctor, eyebrows raised high.

Other unforgettable experiences during the long hospital
siege came from hearing my occasionally profane but often loud
uncle, whose room was just down the hall. We didn't visit often,
but the crusty old cattleman—reportedly a true master of the
cattle business—was much in evidence late at night. Instead
of calling for a nurse, he would summon his wife. Grady Pruet
would call for his wife in the same tone and decibel level that
he would have used to call up a herd. Well after visiting hours
but usually before most of us had dropped off to sleep, the
entire sixth floor would hear Grady call, "Dinnnkkkk!!!!" I
don't know when or even *if* Dink came, but somehow it was
comforting to know that he was quickly satisfied and that she
was probably there.

Dink could not spend all her time in the hospital with
Grady. Often she and two other aunts from the "old home
place" for the Texas Pruets, the village of Putnam located thirty

miles east of Abilene, would visit both Grady and me. I speak
with reverence when I talk of my Putnam relatives, the closest
of whom are all now united in a higher home. There are no
replacements in our society for that breed of country folk. Then,
however, they were full of life and the kind of stories that
defy description. If I could only reproduce—complete with
accent, facial expression, and voice tone—some of the tales that
Dink and Reba told about their elder sister, Lillie; or how
they described certain domino-playing antics of Ellison and
my other Putnam uncle, Homer; or of the serious problems
encountered in one of their fishing expeditions—if I could do
it, I would transmit a fragment of true Americana. Such was
part of my heritage in the hospital.

One other specific example of "humor in the hospital" happened well into my second month in Hendricks. As described
earlier, things were not going well as far as recovery was concerned. A feeling of numbness had spread well upward from its
belt-around-the-stomach beginning. I was uneasy, to say the
least, as shown that day by my question to Dr. Regenio: "What
will happen if the numbness moves further upward to my
heart?"

"Nothing," Dr. Regenio replied. "MS doesn't kill."

Without expanding on the possibilities, I thought, "It's sure
done enough already. I can only trust that you are right about
that next step!"

Soon after the doctor left, my steady stream of company, in
addition to my ever present Myra Sue, began for the morning.
By now there were of course enough chairs in the room to
handle all visitors. Aunt Lillie, one of my dearest aunts, swept
into the room, carrying a large brown paper bag full of fresh
green beans. She explained carefully that she had caught a ride
from Putnam with Dink today especially to bring a "few beans"
from the garden to Myra Sue. Of course the beans had to be
snapped before cooking; so both she and willing wife settled
down there in the hospital room to the job of "snapping beans,"
smoothly blending vocal and vegetable sounds.

Unexpectedly, Dr. Regenio, accompanied by nurse and the

infamous syringe, popped back into the room. He announced, "We need another 'spinal.' Everybody out, please."

Myra Sue left as requested, but Aunt Lillie settled a little lower in her chair, fully preparing to watch what this little doctor was going to do to her favorite nephew. "After all," she must have thought, "I'm seventy-three years old, aren't I? I've got another nephew who is a doctor, don't I? Doesn't that make me some kind of an expert?"

I thought nervously to myself, "The last thing I need at a time like this is someone to distract the guy that is sticking me with that superneedle!!"

"Aunt Lillie!" I said, with perhaps more sharpness than the queen of the Lottie Moon Christmas offering from the First Baptist Church of Putnam, Texas, expected, "You have to take your beans and *go!*"

Funny? Ridiculous? Perhaps it doesn't seem so to you; nor, I admit, did it to me at the time it happened. Now, however, it brings me a broad smile whenever I think of it.

The point behind all these stories is simply to emphasize the value of a sense of humor in a long hospital experience. Laughter even to one on a sick bed comes from person-to-person exchanges whenever both people relax, actually look for the lighter side, and somehow postpone more serious moments. Put another way, this means cultivating a healthy sense of humor, regardless of health itself.

Lack of a realistic outlook? Overlooking the seriousness of the situation? My answer to both these questions is an emphatic *no!* Humor is a positive force that softened my sharp edges, deflated my ego, and sustained me in long battles.

Sustaining forces such as humor, friends, relatives—even prayer—were stretched very near to the breaking point by the last half of July. Progress toward the kind of health that I used to take for granted—the ability to function physically and to move freely—was as elusive as promise for the future. As a matter of fact, fast-moving events during the last two weeks of July 1963 launched me on a "quest for the best" and also stripped me of sustaining confidence.

3

Quiet Desperation—
Experiences and Answers

How can one adequately describe those times when patience wears very, very thin; when prayers seem to bounce back from the ceiling; when hope is simply a four-letter word with no meaning; when quiet desperation pleads for expression? With great difficulty and hesitation, that's how.

After nearly two months in the same room in the same hospital with the same doctors and the same nurses treating the same symptoms, there should have been some change for the better. Not so in this case, however. My confinement designed supposedly to counteract MS symptoms had developed into a mentally comfortable capsule, insulated from the real world. But the treatment brought no improvement physically.

The realities of the outside world, as well as the obvious problems of our leasing company now without its manager, were not really neglected or forgotten. Rather those facts were somehow postponed. Without specifically planning how it could be so, I unconsciously reshaped and delayed daily realities, as if life and problems in Midland could be frozen, packaged, and then marked "Hold Until Opened" when I returned.

Impending events soon made me realize that life continues "in spite of" instead of "waiting patiently for."

Unexpectedly, my three associates in our leasing company came briskly into my room that hot July day about two hours before lunch. Since I had missed hearing from them except by reported greetings from mutual friends, I was very pleased at their coming—but just a tiny bit apprehensive. After they warmly greeted Myra Sue and passed on news from their wives in Midland, the conversation slowed appreciably. I was well acquainted with their custom of not discussing business in front of their women (typical among most of us, I'm afraid); so I shooed friend wife from the room.

I am sure that I began by chattering (with some misgivings) about my diagnosis and the chances for an early recovery—realizing all the while that the only thing I could actually demonstrate was a well-learned proficiency to lie in a hospital bed. Shifting subjects, I quickly asked about general news regarding oil activity in West Texas, and then about particular news concerning our leasing company.

Each of the three answered my general questions and then told about what he had been doing, about certain major leases that our company had added, about questions our secretary had been getting from customers about my absence, as well as greetings from our banker.

Our leasing company was a firm which bought any kind of equipment that a customer wanted, ranging from a typewriter to a drilling rig—and then leased (rented) it to him for long periods. My job was to negotiate the lease, arrange financing, and supervise collections. My secretary and I were the only full-time employees.

As an equal stockholder with my associates, I was pleased to hear of the continued growth of our young company. As a matter of fact, I had always thought of myself more as an owner-organizer than as an employee. As the "hired" general manager, however, I was quietly deflated that it had done so well without me.

After we had exhausted all conversational topics, the group smoothly shifted to a line of thought that reintroduced me to reality. It was done so adroitly that *much later* I could admire their skill. At the time however, my mood changed from deflation to quiet desperation. After expressing concern about the cost of my long hospital stay,·L. D. glanced at his companions for affirmed, well-rehearsed support and said, "Ronald, we've missed you in Midland, but you understand that we had to arrange for someone to handle your job—temporarily, of course."

Smiling, I replied with an affected assurance, "Sure, L.D., I understand. I'm sorry that I've been sidetracked for so long. It sure sounds like things are going well anyway. Let me say this, though. I'm not going to be in the hospital much longer, even though I can't predict the exact date I'll be back in the saddle."

Bob then assumed the role of spokesman after nodding at L. D. and Harold. He quickly said, "Ronald, that's one of the reasons we all came to see you. Looking at all the uncertainties and the terrific hospital expenses you're running up, we have agreed to buy your stock in the company." Hurriedly, he went on, "Your worries about hospital expenses would sure be eased in case you go ahead and sell. I'm sure that we could agree on a fair market price."

I am certain that a blank look came on my face, hardly hiding my abrupt shock of learning that competitive life does indeed go on, in spite of hospital interruptions. There probably was no intended cruelty and *may* have been little greed on the part of these, my friends and business associates. Realistically, they were only protecting our substantial investment in a new business.

My considerable uneasiness at their stated "offer" to buy me out probably came first from believing that "all would be well" without a contribution of effort from me to the firm (head-in-the-sand approach), second from my sudden recollection of "horse-trading" techniques where two or more band together for a trading advantage over a third party (the exercise of which all three were masters), and last, from the realization that there was no permanence (perhaps little remaining life) in my job or investments. "Considerable uneasiness" drastically understates how much I was really worried.

I quickly told them—probably almost stammered, "What you

all are suggesting is a real surprise to me. I hadn't ever considered selling out! Don't worry, I'll be back soon. I want to
take up where I left off."

Almost as soon as I got the words out, my business partners
said their "So longs" and then left to return to west Texas and
the bright sunshine.

The sharp spur which I had just received threatening my
business position, my very job, did not give me the kind of
jolt that aided improvement. Neither, as a matter of fact, were
there any predictions from my doctors when I asked them later
about when I might be able to go back to work.

About mid-afternoon Myra Sue said to her glum husband,
"I've been talking to your doctor cousin about how you're
getting along. After we talked awhile, I asked him about getting advice from other specialists. Do you know what he said?
He told me that if he were in your place, he would go somewhere else—maybe even Mayo Clinic." Then she firmly said,
"I agree with him. I think we ought to go to Mayo's."

Instead of agreeing with the "why?" I looked at the "why
not?" Sputtering about the costs and means of getting to
Rochester, Minnesota, where Mayo's is, plus the problem of
getting into the clinic if I got there, plus the difficulty of paying
the clinic charges, I protested the whole idea. But to no avail.

Barriers I raised, either real or imagined, were to that determined woman of mine nothing more than things to get around
or push aside. We talked and reviewed just how well I was
doing. In a few minutes I reassessed my "nonrecovery" to date
and reluctantly agreed to try to go.

When we agreed to act, barriers began to fall.

We began by brainstorming about the various ways for a
bed-bound patient to get from Abilene to Rochester. Car?
train? plane? Sure, that's it! A reasonably large private plane
was really the only practical way to get there. The catch was
that I didn't have such an airplane, nor did my partners. Telephone calls to other possibilities in Midland resulted in dead ends.

One more long shot—a call to my dad (who didn't have a
plane either) produced results. He was able to arrange through

one of his nephews for the use of a private plane, complete with pilot, to fly us north. My breath caught sharply when I learned that the plane would pick me up *the very next day!*

Arrangements made that same evening by my Abilene doctors included my admission to the Mayo Clinic, hospital reservations in Rochester, an ambulance to meet me, and a motel room for Myra Sue. Almost unbelievably, in less than twenty-four hours after we had decided to act, the plane carrying my wife and me landed 1,200 miles from home, and I was loaded into an ambulance which headed five more miles from the airport to St. Mary's Hospital in Rochester. When I needed it most, the decision to *act* rather than worry about the forces that might keep me from acting opened avenues to change stalled conditions.

It is difficult to describe all my feelings when I checked into that huge hospital in a strange city. I was awed by its size and even impressed by the printed brochure telling me about its equipment and history. I was subdued at the thought of being a patient in the internationally famous Mayo Clinic. Probably my first down-to-earth thought came when I realized that the clinic doctors *and* all their knowledge would come to me in that room, since I couldn't come to them.

As to the advice they would give me, however, I know that I expected something like sparkling words from a "higher plane" that would change the whole picture. First, I hoped for a different diagnosis. In any event, I was confident of a quick plan to cure what was the matter. Yes, I expected a man-supplied miracle, even though none had been promised. Nor did I find their examination routine substantially different from what I had been going through for the last two months.

Mayo's answer to those soaring hopes began on the very night I checked in. A white-smocked intern dismissed Myra Sue and launched into that *thrice* repeated summary of my medical history. The next day included repeats of earlier tests—including a spinal. The following day included a visit by a squad of seven —count them—seven doctors at one time, all of whom specialized in neurological disease. Then followed delays upon more delays followed by inaction. As a matter of fact, the effects of the whole Mayo consultation can best be described by telling about events and emotions on Monday, the sixth day in that efficient but loneliest of hospitals in Rochester.

I was, by nature, self-reliant and did not normally need help in controlling my feelings. Furthermore, the "stark lonesome plains of the West" was where I lived then, and some might say that therefore I was "trained" to endure. Never *anywhere,* however, have I felt more alone than on that particular day in that hospital. Sure, nurses were bustling about; orderlies were available; doctors passed by; and Myra Sue came when visiting hours allowed. Yet this was not a normal day, because I had been promised—since last week—that the multiple sclerosis specialist, Dr. Goldstein, would come. He would personally give me the diagnosis of Mayo Clinic. Waiting for him, the part of me that thinks and fears, Ronald himself, was battling the kind of loneliness that invades the inner rooms where patience usually protects.

I realize now, in looking back, what I didn't understand then. Jesus once told His disciples who were being threatened with physical harm, "In your patience, possess ye your souls" (your emotions, intellect, and inner being). My patience was gone. I was soon to experience what happens to one without it.

As the long tedious day dragged on, there was no evidence of Dr. Goldstein. He seemed nothing more than a promise and only a vague one at that. As I lay there in that narrow room, seven desolating emotions came trooping in, much the same fashion as the seven specialists did last week. In came loneliness, frustration, doubt, fear, pessimism, despair, hopelessness—seven negative emotions clamoring for pieces of my soul. Each got at least a part.

Finally, well after the evening meal, came the long-awaited visit from the "Last Word" in human expertise in neurological disease. The small, balding doctor was quite calm and, to my mind's eye now, expressionless. He began by saying, "Our diagnosis confirms what your doctors in Abilene thought—you have multiple sclerosis."

In a small voice, I said, "Dr. Goldstein, I was hoping that you could have found something else. But as you see, I am in pretty rough shape now. What can we do to work back to where I was before, physically?"

"Mr. Pruet, in view of your condition, recovering what you used to have is quite impossible. But we have used a program for some of our MS patients that come to the clinic that has sometimes met with some success. Frankly, I don't know what it will do for your case."

He paused for a moment as if considering whether I was "worthy" of being anointed with the benefits of his experience. Then he said, "Before we could consider beginning that treatment procedure, you must understand the possibilities that you face. First of all, there will not necessarily be any change in your condition. Second, there are often severe, undesirable side effects from this medical treatment."

"Side effects, doctor?" I questioned quietly.

"Yes, bleeding ulcers are not at all uncommon. More patients, however, develop diabetes. I mention these things, of course, only as possibilities. Even so, we would not begin this regimen unless you understood the dangers."

"Doctor Goldstein, I've been under treatment for two months without any favorable predictions. Surely you can give some encouragement about your Mayo Clinic plan."

"Well, Mr. Pruet, there is a chance that some improvement would develop. Frankly though, you will be fortunate to make it to a wheelchair." (I tell you this peculiar fact: Myra Sue was there and swears that she heard that last statement. My own mind refuses to "copy" that I ever heard it.)

"But what about my life span, doctor? Will MS shorten my life?"

"It will probably shorten it a little. There is a chance though that you will live near to your normal life expectancy." (Another human peculiarity—I heard this last statement, but Myra Sue doesn't remember it at all.)

"Is there any reason that I couldn't take the Mayo treatment in Abilene instead of here?"

"Mr. Pruet, we prefer to supervise the plan directly. However, we *could* send the prescribed treatment with you if you prefer. If your doctors have any questions, please have them call me."

After perfunctory well wishes, Dr. Goldstein vanished.

The night that followed was the most desolate in my life. My last hope for a reprieve from MS had been replaced minutes earlier by dismal predictions for my future by an expert in his field. Visions of my life as a bed-bound cripple—possibly a human vegetable—became so real, so solid, that my active past seemed to be only imagination. All I could forsee was either complete dependence or an early end. The seven desolating emotions took full possession of my soul.

As a response, I cried.

My wife comforted.

All of the human help that either of us had that night came from the single telephone call which we made. The answering "angel," the one who flew us here a single week before, heard our call for help. He agreed to pick Myra Sue and me up tomorrow to return to Abilene.

Visiting hours were over, and separate emotional battles continued through the night for both Myra Sue and me.

The pale green walls of my room in St. Mary's seemed even colder and less hospitable that night. Bounding from wall to wall were echoes of loneliness, self-pity, and all the mental anguish that one can inflict on himself.

Each wall seemed to whisper to me in consecutive order, "You're a long way from home, and I offer you little hope." "Some patients with what you have never get up at all." "Some as ill as you never leave this room." The last wall, the one with the small Madonna hanging near the bed, said nothing at all.

Myra Sue told me much later that in her motel room she had cried, tossed, prayed, and then pleaded. Her total sleeping time? None. Comfort from my reaction? None. Comfort and assurance from the Bible? Yes. Instructions to early Christians became so real to her that night that they became a personal promise. Paul had written, "Your faith should not stand in the wisdom of men, but in the power of God."

As for me, I cannot claim that the peace that dissolved my despair came because of *recognizable* answers to prayers of my own—and, believe me, I prayed. Somehow though, desperation turned into hope by the next morning. Perhaps it was all because of answered intercessory prayer. Perhaps it was because today we would be flying south. Perhaps it was because of a natural tendency to bounce back. Perhaps it was because I believed the Mayo prescription would be a winner for me. All I know is this: For whatever reason or combination of reasons, we both felt hopeful, even though nothing had actually changed during the night.

In addition to hope, one thing more was strengthened in my outlook. *Determination*—call it self-will if you like or call it answered prayer if you prefer—became a strong part of me. It became very clear to me that God did not intend that I lay passively in the hospital waiting for desired changes. My part was simply *to try to recover* with every ability, gift, blessing, advice, medical aid, assistance—everything that had been given me.

As we litted off the ground in our borrowed "angel" about midmorning toward Abilene, my spirits soared. Our short stay in Rochester had not been so painful because of any lack of care, either in or out of the hospital. My misery had been magnified by nothing more than my emotions. But, oh, those emotions!

It was probably *my* fault of course. I had traveled with Myra Sue in an airplane before, and I should have told her not to drink that coffee. (Actually, she has been known to have the same trouble traveling in a car to the grocery store.) She had dramamine for air sickness, but our trusty "angel" in no way ·had provisions for female bladder relief. As time stretched to three, then four, then f-i-v-e hours of continuous flying, Myra Sue's vital s-t-r-e-t-c-h reached its limit. She had kept me informed, and her repeated grimaces of genuine pain led me to ask the pilot to land first in Wichita Falls—in Texas but still thirty minutes from home.

Upon seeing that same pilot years later, he told me that he still remembered the expressions of relief that he saw on both our faces when she got back on the plane in a few minutes— mine for returning to Texas, hers for both that cause and also for the more obvious reason of an unscheduled relief stop.

That night I checked into the "new wing" at Hendricks— the same hospital, mostly different nurses, the same doctors, but with a different medicine plan. The Mayo Clinic approach which I delivered to my doctors involved a series of massive shots of drugs called steroids. The Mayo prescription was faithfully administered and carefully watched from the very beginning. After all, my doctors were also cautioned about probable side effects, in even more detail than Dr. Goldstein told me personally.

All right, what about the actual side effects that came? There was never an indication at all of diabetes. There were no bleeding ulcers. As a matter of fact, the only noticeable side effect from the whole treatment was a retention of body fluid, which was easily counterbalanced by a daily use of a foul-tasting purple medicine.

And the possible improvement? In less than a week I was able to move muscles which had been unresponsive. First there was an improvement in taking exercises while lying in bed, then in moving about the room, then—giant step—up and down the hall outside my room. I remember well the instructed walking exercises in the hallway—step on alternate squares of the tiles. Late evening visitors in that wing must have wondered when they saw that awkward six-footer seemingly playing hopscotch up and down the hall in his pajamas.

Yes, in spite of earlier fears, "recovery" was well on the way within two weeks after beginning the treatment program. Furthermore, along with physical improvement, came healing of my spirits—my outlook for the future. And, you know, this healing of my mental outlook—the "unseen" part of my affliction with MS—was just as important, actually maybe even more so, than correcting the physical effects of the illness. Really, the unseen part of me "hurt" the most when I was in the hospital.

My spirits were nursed from a number of specific sources during those weeks in August. What about that homemade peach ice cream that June, my sister-in-law, often brought! Too, I couldn't leave out the regular gifts of male companionship from Dub Orr over a chessboard. I seldom won but always enjoyed the game. Put it all together, the demonstrated love from family and friends that was given to me during trying times speeded my recovery in spirit just as much as the daily shots aided my physical improvement.

As recovery accelerated, I will never forget the first time in nearly three months that I got dressed to go outside. Shaving had become less difficult. (Most men take for granted how "easy" it is to *stand* in front of the mirror to shave—sometimes it's *not* easy for some). Choosing clothes to wear, however, was simple because Myra Sue brought only one set to the hospital. The day was a typical August scorcher. Rather than hiding from the sun, though, I absorbed both inwardly and outwardly every ray of sunshine I could find when I went outside. There was something about the Texas sunshine that seemed to purge all that ailed me. Then I walked all the way to the front sidewalk and back!!

Toward the end of August, the simple act of walking became more and more a pleasure. The only admonition I had from my doctors was to walk only until I was "tired" but not "fatigued." (I never did learn to judge properly that point where tiredness stops and fatigue begins.) By the end of about three weeks I was walking with strength (but little agility) to "distant" goals as far as two whole blocks away. I say "two whole blocks" with tongue in cheek, not because that distance is so much to be admired, but because it was far enough to get me to my leasing company chores at work in Midland.

Yes, after three months instead of a "couple of days for a checkup," the Ronald Pruet family returned home. On September 1, Myra Sue, the three kids who had funneled back to Abilene, and I drove back to Midland. I could safely drive the car, so I began working again immediately—a half day at first and then gradually to a "normal" full-time schedule. Give them credit too—my partners *did* seem glad to have me back, and at no time later did they specifically bring up "buying me out" again.

But what and how does one feel after supposedly "recovering" from an incurable disease? Frankly, I knew in my heart that I was in what doctors call a "remission," the "go" stage of this come-and-go disease. A complete recovery I did *not* have. Within a few months, however, I walked well enough to hide the crippling episode that I had been through, although I did not have enough agility or endurance to play tennis or golf. I could ride a bicycle, drive a car, and "run" with the kids in the yard (at the four-year-old son's speed). I had come a long way! For that I was truly thankful.

It did not take long before business drive and personal ambition were nearly as important to me as they ever were, and, believe me, they *were* important. An early return to intense competition in the business and professional world was probably caused by two different factors. First, I felt a need to show my hard-driving business associates that I had lost relatively little because of MS; second, I had always possessed a strong motivation to succeed in the task at hand.

All in all, things were going well for us. Myra Sue began teaching the fourth grade, a position she filled admirably. The kids were happy.

Financial worries were eased when insurance picked up the major costs of all my hospital expenses. That simple statement masks yet another "coincidence" regarding a random decision on my part—to sign up for group insurance about six weeks before I went to the hospital.

Yes, life in Midland seemed to settle into something like a routine once more. I suppressed negative possibilities about my crippling, unpredictable disease, and then resumed nearly every activity.

All this—and yet I was vaguely uneasy. I sensed, and perhaps unconsciously feared, what the future might hold for me and my family.

4

Changing Directions

Talk about a complete surprise! It was a bolt to the bald prairie all the way from the town with no strangers. The time was the evening of the first Sunday in January; the setting my house in Midland. I was relaxing in front of the fireplace, enjoying the crackling fire. Myra Sue and the two older boys rattled the dishes in the kitchen after the evening meal, and the youngest was quiet for a change, mainly because his brothers were busy. And then the telephone rang. It was my mother and dad.

After we exchanged the conventional greetings and exclaimed "how much we enjoyed the nice Christmas gifts," dad took over the talk from Ranger. I could tell by his change in tone and speed that he shifted his talking gear from "conversation" to "well-rehearsed speech."

Before I could decide whether the news would be good or bad, he quickly said, "Let's see now—it's been about sixteen months since you got out of the hospital, hasn't it? You tell us that you are getting along all right with that leasing business too, don't you?"

Then without waiting for my response, he continued, "Your mother and I have been doing a lot of thinking about your situation there. Of course we want things to work out well for your family; so we have something that you and Myra Sue ought to consider."

With hardly a pause for breath, he blurted, "We think that you should think about going back to school. That route looks like the sensible way to prepare yourself for a better job. We know it would be expensive to go back to college with your family, but we've looked at the whole picture. We're prepared to help with the expenses if you decide to go."

My silence after he finished accurately showed how stunned I was.

Because he said it almost without stopping, I could tell that it was a carefully planned speech. Because of his tone, I could also tell that they meant it.

The first thing I did was to tell him how flat-footed his suggestion caught me. Then I started listing some of the obvious shortcomings of their idea: First, it had been nearly sixteen long years since I had graduated from Texas Tech. Second, I was satisfied doing what I was doing. After all, I didn't just have a job, I was part owner.

Dad simply said that his idea deserved some thought on my part, and that a better future might be in prospect. I was intrigued at the idea of being a student again but was also convinced by my own arguments against the practicality of a thirty-four-year-old father of three—with MS—going back to college. I thanked them again and said I would think about it seriously.

My thinking about that possible change, however, was just part of the question. Sure, if I went back to school, it would be *I* who had to perform. But *I* would not be the only one affected. Myra Sue and the boys would change from a businessman's family to a student's family. Think about it—there's a great deal of difference.

As a matter of fact, there had been some pressures from my business partners. I could never quite tell if the vibrations I felt were intentional on their part or incidental to the business. It was not so much *what* I was doing as general manager or even *how* I was doing it. Rather the pressure came from feeling how closely my associates watched me as to the quantity of physical work I did—a perpetual assessment, so to speak, of my physical qualifications. And I never knew just what they thought the physical qualifications were. Eight hours seemed to call for ten.

My wife and I were convinced after many evenings of considering the effects of dad's proposal on our family, our life style, our future—indeed, our whole life's direction—that this decision was really too important to handle without help. Wise King Solomon had the advice that we leaned on. He said something like this: "Trust in the Lord with all your heart. Don't depend on your own understanding. In all your problems trust Him and He will direct your paths." To us that sounded like good advice.

Actually, that phone call from the folks about school was something remarkable in itself. Never had I talked with them about more education; indeed, I had never even thought of trying for a master's or doctorate. When I graduated back in the Dark Ages (1949), my total ambition centered only on work—not more education.

"But then again...now is another time," I pondered to myself. The thoughts that followed became an almost perpetual debate between "Status Quo" on one side and "More Education" on the other. "S.Q.," whose nature was normally more comfortable for me, was an expert rationalizer. Points on his side included the fact that I had a job I enjoyed, associates who were congenial even though somewhat demanding, part ownership in a business I helped organize, and a measure of recognition in the community. "Opportunity" was merely an acquaintance then. As yet we were not close friends.

Then "M.E." would speak up with a challenging note. He would claim that college as an undergraduate had not been overly difficult for me, that intellectual challenge would be stimulating, that opportunities in business would be magnified with more education. Finally, he would play his trump card: there was no guarantee that another attack would not lay me low someday.

"If that ever happened again with the same job in Midland," he would ask, "where would you be with those 'patient' partners of yours?" I couldn't answer.

The results of the debate at least convinced me to do my part in cracking the doors to college. As a matter of fact, I grudgingly decided to talk to an industrial engineering professor at Texas Tech around the middle of January. Since I was a registered professional engineer, he was quite receptive and encouraging. One indication became apparent: the door might swing open if I pushed a little harder. He cautioned, however, that the GRE (graduate record examination) must be taken and passed before anyone can be admitted to graduate school. Another barrier.

It was about this time that several alternatives became clearer. I had been working closely with banks for about four years. Because I enjoyed that contact as well as participating in the business world, I realized that more engineering education was not for me. Yes, business held my interest more. Furthermore, *if* I were to try graduate work in Texas, the University of Texas in Austin would be my choice because of the reputation of its business school.

About the same time, Myra Sue and I agreed that we should not make a change unless *four* doors would swing wide open. After all, we said, if our prayers were heard, and the Lord was directing our path, the change would be an invitation instead of a problem. These four doors (barriers every one) were, first of all, a favorable interview with an outstanding finance professor; second, a good score on the GRE; third, sale of our home in Midland; and last, sale of my stock in our leasing company for an adequate price. Only favorable action on all four barriers would be the sign of the guidance we sought.

Naturally, I don't mean to imply that we had answers to prayer that were unique. Furthermore, I don't infer that I challenged God to hand me specific listed gifts as signs that He heard us. Nor do I imply that I expected to receive without giving my own best efforts. I do not hesitate to claim, however, that He supplied what I lacked when I needed it most. Furthermore, I believe that He had, even *has*, a plan for me and mine, though I don't yet fully understand it. He does listen to earnest prayer, because I'd seen it happen before in the hospital. In summary, perhaps I should only claim that we *did* pray.

The first hurdle, the GRE exam, was a "biggie." I remember studying a book of sample questions which were supposed to be representative of the two-part test, the verbal and mathematical sections. I had signed up—very quietly of course— to take the exam at nearby Odessa in late February. As the time to take the quiz finally came, I filed into the room with about fifty younger "students," convinced that the only thing about me that was sharp were the pencils that I brought. After all, if those questions that I had been studying were good samples, I was *assured* of only a dismal grade that might admit me to the Bug Tustle Business College.

I did my best and left in a couple of hours with a slightly lower level of confidence than I had when I started. (Hard to imagine but true!)

In a few weeks I called the School of Business of Texas University and asked to speak with a professor in the finance department. I knew no one at the school, did not know about my GRE score, and was only seeking a weekend appointment to talk generalities about the MBA (master of business administration) program there. Some smart secretary suggested that I talk with Dr. Charles Prather. In our conversation he did not hesitate to ask me down to Austin for a Saturday morning meeting in late March.

After a couple of weeks with my companions, Foreboding and Uncertainty, I decided to keep the appointment. Friday afternoon, after Myra Sue had finished teaching and I had wound up the week's work, we pointed the station wagon southeast toward Austin and headed out. When Saturday morning came, I wondered what on earth I was doing down there. A spring track meet, the Texas Relays, had just about exhausted the accommodations in and near Austin, and so our motel was not what would be called "choice." It seemed that we looked all over "the 40 acres" that morning to find the man I came to see, but finally I knocked on his office door.

My first contact with a Texas University professor was a most pleasant surprise. Here was a man at peace with himself. His office, with books lining the wall, and with pictures, awards, and degrees much in evidence, reflected comfort, confidence, and accomplishment. Dr. Prather, I later learned, was about two years away from retirement and was considered nationally to be a distinguished author and professor. When I told him that I was considering graduate school, he welcomed me as if Texas University (with about 40,000 students then) actually needed such a student as I.

I had made up my mind earlier that I would tell no one at any school about multiple sclerosis and me; so Dr. Prather's invitation to graduate school was not based on sympathy. Mainly, he tried to convince me that an "old man," going on thirty-six could make it and benefit. I was favorably impressed, but not quite convinced about giving up a bank book for a school book.

About two weeks later in the mail I got an envelope with a window in it that didn't include a bill. It was the score of my GRE. I was most pleasantly surprised that I had a combined score that was well above the required grade for admittance to the MBA program at Texas University. The score was high enough to get me in but, not surprisingly, low enough to remind me that I was several steps below the genius level. But at the same time, I recalled that sixteen years ago my college grades weren't at the genius level either.

That score and the favorable interview with Dr. Prather led to the next "step" or "stop," whichever it was to be, namely, the sale of our house. The outlook for that project can be surmised by the following facts. One house in our neighborhood in Midland had been advertised for sale well over one year, with no sale to date. The home we were living in had been vacant for about the same length of time before we bought it seven years earlier. Real estate in Midland then was not going "like hotcakes," and believe me, I knew because I had been a real estate salesman (part time) a few years earlier. I still felt secure in advertising my house for sale bècause of the slow market on the one hand and the game of musical houses that Midlandites customarily played on the other hand. Selling a house did not necessarily announce a planned move from town.

The surprise in this case came when a real estate agent brought a prospective buyer to the house. She announced that her client liked the house, had the money, and wanted to move in by June 1. Simply put, things moved like clockwork. It seemed as if I had stepped on a greased slide and was literally propelled to the fourth door—selling my business interest.

In April of '64, the previous year, I had sold the coin operated laundry that I had installed and operated for six years. Frankly, the machines had cried for someone with more energy (and patience) than I to maintain them. Now, however, in April 1965, my task was to sell my quarter interest in our leasing company—a much more formidable proposition.

I called a breakfast stockholders' meeting, as was our custom in discussing various leases under consideration. This time at our meeting, I told my associates that I wanted to sell out. They were completely surprised when I told them that I was thinking about going back to college. My partners were not overly impressed with value to be gained from more education, nor did they at first believe that more education was my real goal. With as much uncertainty that I had in getting to where I was, I couldn't blame them! Even so, I gave one month's notice and said, "I intend to enroll at UT in about five weeks."

Later that same day we brought up the question of price. That subject could have been the one that turned the whole picture around. We had no trouble, however, reaching a figure that was agreeable to both sides. As a matter of fact, we were so congenial that I agreed to represent "our" company as an agent in Austin.

With that, the die was cast for me and mine to become UT and Austin schoolboys. All four doors had been opened and opened wide. Even now I look back with awe at the speed of the change, the finality of the move, and the effects of following the path that my Guide opened for us.

Really, however, I had seen before, in our "decision" to go to Mayo's how smoothly a shift of direction goes when I *rested* in His hands. Sure, from January to June I could have lost sleep about how I might perform as a student again, and worried about my home and stock sale prices, plus the dollar-costs of the proposed move. But I simply trusted that it would turn out right after I did my part, and the whole change moved with clockwork precision.

In the second week of June 1965, I was plunged into mysteries of such subjects as accounting and finance. A new language had to be learned to cover the shift from the seat-of-the-pants accounting that I had actually used in my firm and the workaday finance of my real business to the textbook approach to the same problems. I soon learned that my instinctive approach was not necessarily the best way to tackle the problems. Certainly it was not the best way to earn my new goal of an "A" in the classroom instead of a "$" in Midland. By the end of that first summer session, however, I had made the necessary shift.

One part of college which I both enjoyed and sometimes reluctantly respected was the stimulation from competing and associating with younger minds. I found that socially I had little in common with them. Intellectually they were often ahead of me, and as to creed and cause, they listened to a different drummer.

Yet in the classroom we had common goals—to learn and achieve. The so-called generation gap was apparent when I considered their way of looking at life, their views of the Vietnam War, and their plans for the future, be it next weekend or next decade. The very least I could say is that it *was stimulating*.

The MBA program at UT called for two years of instruction in varied business subjects such as marketing, management, accounting, finance, and statistics. When I was an engineering student at Texas Tech between sixteen and twenty years earlier, we derisively looked down on business students with the stated slur, "Run and play for a BBA." I can testify that the program that I went through at Texas University was a different proposition from what I had imagined earlier to be fun and games in business education.

Time passed with surprising speed, and I found myself completing my MBA thesis and degree in the summer of 1967, right on schedule. Probably the only twinge of looking back during this period came from phantasizing after Midland friends came to see us in Austin. It seemed as if each had just turned (sold) a profitable deal or started a new company that promised large profits. I could counter their impressive business progress only by reporting that I made three "A's" and two "B's" last semester. I sometimes was consoled when some of these friends in the mainstream said, "Someday, I just might do what you're doing." Some really meant it.

With an MBA behind me, I reached other crossroads. Looking for a job in industry was one choice; continuing my education to the "terminal degree" (collegese for a Ph.D.) was the other. A very interesting possibility developed when I explored my chances for a doctorate in ecoonmics.

"With that degree," I said to myself, "I could get a job in a bank or a large oil company." I weighed what would be required of me, checked the dollar problems, and decided not only to continue my education but also to make the switch from business to economics. My chief economics professor said there was a lot more theory in economics than in business, but I had enjoyed courses that I had taken. Too, I believed that the broader view backed by sound reasoning would have wider application.

My next two years involved accelerated studies, wider reading, and exposure to ideas that were novel to me. I became very well acquainted with such subjects as micro and macro economics (the view of one firm for the first and a study of the whole economy for the second), economic history, as well as money and banking. Though I had doubts that I would be attracted to them if ever I had met them personally, I examined the thinking of such varied men as Adam Smith, John Maynard Keynes, Thorstein Veblen, Karl Marx, and many others. My viewpoint was broadened even further as I added the concepts of an economist to my earlier educational and professional experiences. During the last year I completed my long dissertation and thus finished the assigned race to the doctorate by August 1969.

When I started the whole program four years earlier, my doctor in Abilene told Myra Sue that school was a mistake and that I would never be able to take the pressure. I actually believe the reverse was true. That is, my consuming interest in completing the program *gave* me added strength, a completely opposite result from being drained by challenging programs.

True to the goal I set from the beginning, none of my professors ever knew of my past illness. I did not miss a day from classes because of the chronic illness. Yes, occasionally there were times when a young professor that I was talking to moved rapidly away down the hall as we talked. Because I didn't stay so close to his heels as other "eager" learners, he might have thought that old Pruet was too proud to follow quickly. The truth was that I was just not nimble enough to keep up.

From the very first day to the end, however, I walked the whole campus, usually with no fatigue. I always parked the car several blocks from wherever I was going—not by choice but because of the mob of students. And yet, I truthfully say that I really had no difficulty in getting around there. The mental strain that bears so heavily on graduate students was there. The pressure of comprehensive examinations as I ended the doctorate studies was there. The broad problems involved in researching, writing, revising, and then enlarging a dissertation to satisfy my committee chairman were there. I truthfully say, however, that all the mental strain, pressure, and problems were carried with only reasonable effort. Every deadline was met.

How was this possible for an old student with MS? Of course the conventional credits belong to my wife and boys, as well as to my folks for their support. Too, one could claim that motivation and determination helped make it possible. Altogether though, the conventional credits as I see them are not enough. From the physical standpoint as well as the mental side, I either mustered—or was given—what was needed to get the job done. After carefully looking at the question, I prefer to believe that the Guide who led me to Austin stayed with me through the whole educational period.

As I approached graduation in mid-1969, I went to the annual winter conventions of economists and the plethora of business organizations. Those meetings serve a dual purpose: first to share—call it "demonstrate to other professors"—knowledge about mathematical points concerning theory and second, to allow approaching graduates and prospective colleges to size up each other. I remember a general lack of enthusiasm when I went to the meeting in November of 1968 because I was still convinced that a job in industry or banking was my goal and destiny. Up to then I had not seriously entertained the possibility of becoming a college professor. After all, unlike other hungry graduate students, I had never taught a single undergraduate class in any subject; nor could I picture myself doing so. My teaching experience had been solely "Sunday school," a teaching level invariably omitted on the usual résumé.

After that first professional meeting was over I became acutely aware of how soon I needed to make a decision about a job— within six months. Furthermore, a better job was supposed to be the main reason for more education in the first place, wasn't it? With a jolt, I realized that I had to actively seek and choose the right place and occupation.

First, of course, I had to resolve the dilemma between industry or banking versus the less familiar but somehow attractive college teaching. Understand that I had credentials for any of the three possibilities—professional engineer in industry, bank officer dealing with leasing companies, or college professor. Making the decision was something I could have done by myself or only within my family. However, my family and I were in our present situation in answer to requested guidance. It seemed logical to request it again, and we did.

By the time the main academic meetings began during the Christmas holidays, I had made up my mind to continue along the path I began four years earlier. For the future, I wanted to be on the *other side* of that professor's desk in *front* of the classroom. Like all the other new Ph.D.'s, I put on a new suit and my best smile for the convention in Chicago. There were well over four rings to the "circus," the first attraction being the room where the different colleges and universities from all over the United States listed in large black books the faculty positions which were open, the second a large basement arena with tables to interview prospective candidates, the third the various rooms in the hotel where serious negotiations between deans and faculty candidates were held, and finally the fourth "ring" was of the various rooms where papers on all sorts of subjects were offered almost continuously for four days.

For just this little time at least, to the crop of new graduates from all over the country this was the "greatest show on earth." The biggest attraction was obviously the room where openings in the job market were listed, as shown by the unmasked seriousness which all of us wore as we scurried to the various books to copy more information. The second step in the interview game was to impress the chosen college representatives, as well as to assess all the particulars of the job at the same time. Shortly after the convention was over, our success as candidates was "graded" by whether or not we received a letter inviting us to visit the school or schools where we had indicated we wanted to teach. Of course the last step involved the campus visit, conference with the faculty there, and then a job offer from the dean.

I played the game the same way all the other candidates played it. Yet I had certain preferences as to the place I was to begin teaching. First, I wanted to live in a small town because Myra Sue and I believed that there are fewer problems in raising a family of three boys in that kind of environment. Second, I wanted to deal with students in a college much smaller than Texas University. Third, the south and southwest regions appealed to us more than other parts of the country. Last and most important, we had to have confirmation from the Guide who leads us.

The University of Mississippi, commonly called Ole Miss, located in Oxford, Mississippi, completely filled the four-part bill. Consequently, I have taught here ever since I graduated in 1969. I can tell you without exaggerating that I feel more peace, more fulfillment, and more accomplishment in what I am doing now than I ever felt as a self-employed petroleum engineer and business man. Could it be that following divine direction is more satisfying in the long run?

PART TWO

Wiggling on the Hook

5

People Parts and Soul Scale

Anyone who decides to be a teacher or professor automatically accepts an obligation to share information and ideas. Little did I realize in 1969 when I began my new occupation how much would be required of a professor to continue to *learn* in order to *teach*. It didn't take me long to find out that every bit of my earlier education and business experience is only a license to study and explain subjects that I am teaching at Ole Miss.

Another real eye-opener came when I recently realized that all of my experience with multiple sclerosis—both past and current—just might be another kind of license or obligation to share information and ideas.

I have told you earlier as well as I know how the personal experiences and emotions which I have had with a chronic disease. As far as "information" is concerned, surely that's more than plenty. As to "ideas" though, there's more to come.

During some fourteen years with MS, two before I knew what it was and twelve since the diagnosis, I have had enough time and inspiration to organize some thinking that seems pretty reasonable to me. I am not really interested in trying to explain those ideas in formal medical or religious terms. Anyway, I've told you so much about me that you know I am not trained as a doctor, psychiatrist, or preacher. You must

know, however, that I have a tiger by the tail (or vice versa).
And I hope you get the feeling that I may have learned a
few things as time has passed.

One thing I have noticed is that there are many more than
a few people who have long-term encounters with serious illness or accidents, usually called "chronic illness." I define the
term chronic illness as "an illness, accident, or war wound whose
symptoms linger or recur for long periods of time, and whose
correction is either unknown, uncertain, or restrictive." How's
that for a formal definition of the kind of interruption that
I will refer to for the rest of this book?

The general idea is that with a chronic illness a fellow may
be out of circulation for a long time. It is *to those people*
who are experiencing an unexpected, long-term interruption
of their life plan and routine as well as *to those people* who
deal with, treat, or just plain love them that I address the rest
of this book. Some of the thoughts and experiences I share
might be helpful.

Let's begin this "idea sharing" thing with a definition of
the basic parts of any person—regardless of age, sex, race,
health, or wealth. Let your mind run free to think of three
things that we all have in common.

The most obvious part, the thing about each of us that can
be identified by sight, hearing, or feeling is his *body*. There's
no argument that when anyone is seriously ill or has an accident,
his body usually bears the first effects. It is the body that hurts
when it is hit or bleeds when it is cut. Nothing to this "idea
sharing" so far, is there?

The second part of all people is identified here as his or her
soul. With the word *soul* I have introduced a part of all people
that cannot be seen, heard, or felt directly. In fact most of
us are a little uncertain about the meaning of the word itself.
A person's soul, as I define the word, includes the mind (the
"thinking part" or intellect) and the emotions (the feelings,
and "passion part").

We should recognize too that this important part of "being"
can, like the body, also be chronically ill. When this happens,

a person's soul is treated by another kind of physician, the psychiatrist. So a person's soul includes the part of us that *knows* he is an individual and *feels* such problems as loneliness, depression, anxiety, discouragement, and hate.

It is also very important that we recognize that the soul part of a person loves, has compassion for others, and hopes.

The third part of every person is his or her *spirit*. This part of "being" is also unseen and, because of general confusion about the concept of what "spirit" really means, has been interpreted many different ways. As I see it, a person's spirit is that part of his being that is eternal. In other words, it is that part of a person which can be identified somewhere as long as time is. I think this third part of us is what makes a person greater than the animals.

A very simple diagram—I call it "People Parts"—shows the way I "see" three things we all have in common.

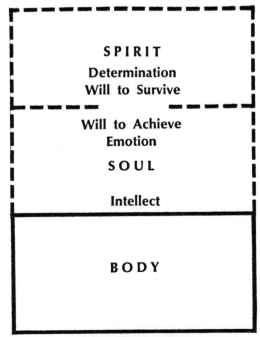

SPIRIT
Determination
Will to Survive

Will to Achieve
Emotion

SOUL

Intellect

BODY

PEOPLE PARTS

Many may not agree about the reality of the spirit or whether it has any relation to chronic illness. All right then—for now let's hold the matter of spirit's influence on chronic illness "constant." (That's the language that economists sometimes use to mean, "We'll deal with that term later.") As for now, I plan to look only at the first two parts: body and soul.

One basic truth about chronic illness—be it physical or mental—is that body and soul affect each other. What I mean by that simple statement is that when the body is seriously ill for a long time and unable to do what is usual and customary, the soul is also affected adversely. In such cases the person's soul usually reacts to daily circumstances differently than it otherwise would.

When the soul is affected by mental illness, extending all the way from lingering melancholy to mental breakdown, the body is almost surely affected too. In this kind of situation the body reacts unpredictably and may even suffer serious damage. Most of us have heard of the medical term *psychosomatic*, which refers to the effects that illness of the soul may have on the body.

All of this definition and discussion is meant to provide a foundation for thoughts about the effects of chronic illness on both the body and soul. Now that it's behind us, let's see if we can organize a few more ideas.

I have seen some studies that tried to measure the effects of a disabling illness. They went into great detail to describe the degree of mobility of the body as measures of disability. For instance, if a fellow could walk, he was graded "one"; if in a wheelchair, he was graded "five." All well and good, I guess, as far as they go.

No mention was made of such an intangible, difficult-to-measure thing as the soul of the one who was disabled. What I am trying to imply is that they missed the most important mark. Body and soul react on each other and usually affect each other as I described earlier. The more important of the two parts is not the body but the soul.

"Wait a minute!" I hear you say. "Do you mean to tell

me it's more important how you *think* you feel than how you actually feel? Don't give me that old mind over body stuff!"

That's a good question and a point well taken. Answering both question and point, here's what I mean. Remember that all I've established is that soul and body interact. What I'm saying is that the soul is the better part to gauge where a patient who is chronically ill actually *is* in relation to where he *could be*. Clearly, I'm not talking like a guru or a faith healer now. I'm talking about the plain old everyday living that goes right on for those people who suffer with a chronic illness.

Maybe this method of measuring "where one is" in chronic illness—call it using the "Soul Scale"—will help to explain what I mean about the importance of the soul.

I visualize five possible levels for the soul of anyone afflicted by a chronic illness.

"Wait a minute!" you say. "I can't *see* the soul."

I answer by asking you to remember that the soul and body affect *each other*. The soul may *lead* the body either up or down. Furthermore, every afflicted person has a good idea where his own soul is. Of this I am almost sure: Whatever the level of anyone's soul, it affects his body.

Now, let's look at those soul levels.

The first of my five levels or gauges of chronic illness is named the *Crashing* level. No, that name was not chosen necessarily to tie it to drinking or drugs. The Crashing level is rock bottom, the time when a man or woman breaks apart emotionally. Surprisingly, I have found more words that describe this time when the soul is literally shattered than for any other emotional level. Think about "desolation," "forsaken," "hopeless," and "despair" as examples.

Imagine with me times and emotions involved when one's mind rejects what seems (or is) actually true concerning his body. Let's say that the body is apparently so damaged that pain and suffering for the rest of his life are all that can be pictured. There is no way to see it otherwise. Or, in other cases the person has suffered a shattering loss of money, business position, or love Life is so bleak that it seems hopeless.

These imaginary examples spotlight times when people might feel completely forsaken and without hope. Their souls could well be pushed to the Crashing level.

The second level, moving upward in my grading scheme, is called the *Quiet Desperation* level. People at this level of chronic illness may be literally hanging by their fingernails to keep from dropping to the level of no hope at all. In this stage rash action is often threatened. In Crashing, such actions are often tried. There is an unmistakable advantage as far as longevity of life is concerned to being in Quiet Desperation instead of Crashing. For such a simple feeling as happiness though, Quiet Desperation is not the place to be. Many of you understand personally; and believe me, I've been there too.

Another way to picture Quiet Desperation is to imagine a person's emotional outlook under extreme anxiety. As best I can remember the emotion, the anxiety of Quiet Desperation is not a constant thing. Instead, it fluctuates according to mood and daily happenings—almost ebbing and flowing like the ocean tides. At its worst the anxiety grows into depression; at its best it goes away. In the long run, however, the person in Quiet Desperation spends most of his time at the low end of the Soul Scale.

The third level is exactly midway in this method of measurement, and it seems proper to call it the *Coping* stage. Coping means fighting a long battle on even terms, sometimes even with success. The individual who is Coping has moved upward from Quiet Desperation to a point where he or she becomes a real person again, one who can do tasks that are worthwhile to himself as well as others. To one who is fighting some types of chronic illness, little things that most people take for granted may become special victories in Coping.

Little tasks like standing while shaving or shopping for family groceries become measurement milestones. Buttoning a shirt, walking out front to get the newspaper, driving the car—all of these little things may become new levels of happiness when one is Coping. Even more, actually *working* on a job—any job—instead of watching others becomes a joy to remember. These listed jobs (or joys) usually cost little effort or thought to healthy people.

For those with chronic illness though, the cost of Coping is often rehearsed planning for every move, practice of the required motions, disciplined effort, and the exercise of strong will. The costs for "little" are thus added and then multiplied. The man or woman at Coping pays these prices, has a glimpse of better things in the future (real or imagined), and feels encouragement in accomplishment.

Without encouragement from *some* accomplishment, those in Coping may go down the Soul Scale instead of higher. Coping by its very name implies that strong effort from the battler is not just required to hold his own—it becomes a way of life.

In his Nobel prize acceptance speech William Faulkner said, "I believe that man will not merely endure; he will prevail!" The name which I have chosen for the next highest level is *Prevailing*. The majesty of Faulkner is necessary to describe some of the victories at this soul level. Lacking that, I will tell you about two examples which speak just as eloquently by their deeds. Perhaps you will understand what I intend to imply for this higher stage.

The first example was someone I knew when I was much younger. He lay in his room at home, completely bed bound and dependent on his parents to move him. Arthritis had taken its toll, beginning for him when he was a teen-ager. Yet the witness he gave to all in Ranger who visited him was cheerfulness, encouragement—and inner strength personified. His attitude was victory rather than defeat.

A second example is a young man who was paralyzed from his neck down by an accident. He is unable to move his legs, has very little control over his arms and even less control of his hands. Instead of giving up, he excelled in college as an undergraduate. What's more, he went to graduate school and completed a Ph.D. in accounting in 1974. But that's not the end of the story—he has begun a full-time career as a college professor.

This man is still paralyzed physically, but his soul has wings.

I watch him daily because he is currently on the faculty here at Ole Miss. I know of the quality of his work, since I served on his doctoral committee. Yes, both of the examples that I have suggested—one deceased and the other quite active—are splendid examples of the Prevailing stage.

The highest level in the Soul Scale is called *Conquering*. As you might imagine, this fifth level is the complete opposite of Crashing. It involves not only a complete cure physically but also complete healing of the soul. Picture complete health at this upper level extreme. All tears are wiped away!

Alas though, you and I know that on this earth that pictured ideal is usually an unattainable goal. The vision of an ancient *Conqueror*—he who has fought and won many battles—seems out of touch with contemporary life. Yet the complete victory of his *Conquering*, though usually unrealized, should be the common goal. I intend that Conquering serves as an ultimate ideal, more than as a way station.

I don't pretend that the five levels that I have just discussed are the only ways to look at "where you are" in chronic illness. But consider the merit of how this gauge works: Look at the simple diagram named "Soul Scale" below. The blank line under

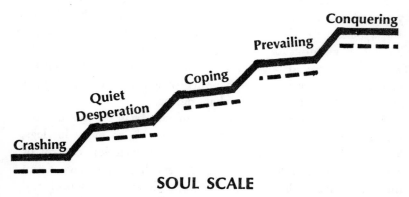

SOUL SCALE

each of the five soul levels is for the name of someone who has had a major interruption. When a specific person is pegged to a specific level, the measurement becomes valuable. Change becomes a "possible" then.

I won't belabor obvious points which can be drawn from my Soul Scale, but you and I can easily see that Prevailing is much to be preferred over Quiet Desperation. But have you noticed that *both* of these levels touch the middle ground that I call Coping? There is no definite fence or barrier separating the five divisions. Instead they blend into each other almost as the colors of the rainbow do.

What this tells me is that while the five levels may indeed be quite distinct, it is also possible for the chronically ill pilgrim to move from one level to another—*either up or down.*

Think about what that last statement implies. We have already agreed that it is better to Prevail than to dwell in Quiet Desperation. If one *can* actually "move" to where it is better, it seems to me that where one who is chronically ill actually "lives" involves two main things: a well-defined choice or goal on his part and then a determined effort to move to the level that appeals to him.

Do you think that solving a serious problem could be so simple? I do.

Now is the time to look at that third part of every person's being. Remember?—I held *spirit* "constant" so we could examine more closely the way body and soul affect each other.

I visualize spirit as being intimately related to, but at the same time different from, the "will" part of soul. I think of spirit as that part of each person that may even add to his being such personality traits as pride and intense curiosity. Furthermore, such basic character strengths as "the will to survive" and "determination to overcome" may have their foundation in the spirit.

But all that I write about a person's spirit is clearly pure speculation, my own ideas that could be *very right* or *very wrong.* As long as you are listening though, I'll throw in my opinion that people's spirits can't move about without the bodies they belong to. Conversely, a *Reader's Digest* condensed book suggests that I might be in error. To clear the air, perhaps I should talk about a certain spirit whom I am better acquainted with.

The spirit to whom I refer is none other than the Holy Spirit, the Comforter that Jesus promised to send when He left.

"Just a big minute now!" I hear you exclaim. "I listened to all that stuff about 'People Parts' and 'Soul Scale,' and I thought you were a little odd. Now you expect me to believe that you *know* the Holy Spirit! You've got some explaining to do—do you think that you're something *special?*"

Absolutely not. If I were special, I'd have told you about it long before this.

All I can say is that I *try* not to be unworthy of the name "Christian." I certainly don't claim to be very good at it! One day I just looked at the promise in the Bible that says the Holy Spirit is available to all who believe.

I believe.

"O.K., then," you persist. "What makes you so sure you know Him?"

That's another good question, but I'm surprised you had to ask it after traveling this far. Here's my answer.

First of all, who do you think is that Guide I have talked about more than once—say, in that trip to Mayo's, or in the decision to go to graduate school? The Holy Spirit.

Next, who do you think comforted, you know—gave peace and confidence—that time I was in Crashing? Or those times when Quiet Desperation had control? The Holy Spirit.

Finally, who do you suppose pointed out those particular passages in the Bible that answered a special need? The Holy Spirit.

Yes—I really should be better acquainted with this Holy Spirit than I actually am. One important thing though—His nearness is not necessarily a function of how *well* I know Him, but just that I *want* to know Him.

"All well and good," you say; "but what's all this Holy Spirit talk got to do with chronic illness?"

I thought you'd never ask! Answering that last question will let me tie all of this together. It just might make sense.

Check back to that Soul Scale diagram again. You see how steep most of those staggered steps are, don't you—particularly

from Crashing to Quiet Desperation (from worst to bad). Because most of the stages are sloping instead of flat, can't you
see too that it's easier to *fall back* instead of *climb up*?

What I'm getting at with the diagrams and discussion is
simply this: You and I need all the help we can get—all the
time—to win the chronic illness battle. Jesus promised the
Holy Spirit for *always* if we ask. And that's not just in church,
but in a hospital and also in everyday problems.

It stands to reason then: If God's Spirit is with my spirit,
nothing is impossible. If He can be with me, He can be with
anyone.

That sounds pretty good, doesn't it?

You know what though? If you are like me (and I suspect
you are if you are truthful), you hesitate to let *anybody* else—
even the Holy Spirit—direct the ways you go. It's really very
hard to turn complete control of old Number One over to
another, especially if you can't see Him.

"After all," you earnestly agree, "how could anyone else
know all that *I've* been through? about what *I* think? about the
best way to solve *my* problems?"

That's exactly the way I see it too!

What's more, during the last twelve years or so, I have fought
the long fight—sometimes well, sometimes poorly—with that
thought in the back of my mind. Most of the time I did it
my way.

As a matter of fact, in *my* efforts to solve *my* problems I
have gone through nearly every common response or reaction
to what has a long-term hold on me. I call those responses
"wiggling on the hook."

Let's explore several of those approaches. Maybe you will
recognize that we just might have more in common than you
thought.

6

I Give Up, and Why Me?

Now, how about some more talk about "wiggling on the hook," my term for responses intended to improve or remove symptoms of chronic illness. I will describe and then classify some of the common ways to "wiggle," and then peg them to the Soul Scale that I told you about. Before I begin though, consider this general background.

You should know that there are two groups of people who are afflicted with chronic illness who for very good reasons do *not* show such responses. The first of those groups (thank You, Lord, for them) is made up of those who are completely cured both physically and mentally of what had been a chronic condition. The second group (God bless their memory) is no longer with us.

That first group of people obviously is not exempt from other problems in the future. They may be considered as special people only in one sense: they have Conquered an interruption that had them under attack so long it was called chronic. Their recovery became simply a milestone in their return and pursuit of "normal activities," whatever that may be.

The second group, a fraternity which I am in no hurry to join, is made of those who have completed a long, usually hard struggle. Yes, just as normal to life as birth is also its natural end after the prescribed number of days.

What's that you ask? "Isn't death a good response in itself to the problems of chronic illness?"

Emphatically—*no!* Because if anyone can't react *daily* to these problems, there is no way that he or she can overcome them. I write this to help the living—not to encourage their early end.

Built into the "spirit-soul" is the will to survive, the ambition to be worthwhile to at least one other, and the desire to give or gain satisfaction. Just because you may be chronically ill doesn't change the importance of those goals that are a natural part of you. Those goals and even more are inside your being. It's your job to become better acquainted with them.

Separate from any other group that I have mentioned before is that very large number of people who are one step away from those with chronic illness. These people are exposed daily to those who are afflicted, but none of this collection is *ill* from the ailment they see so often. Some of this large group dedicate nearly every activity to caring for loved ones; others to treating their symptoms; still others to researching for causes and cures. In contrast, there are probably others who *flee* from reminders of illness in people they care for. All of these people react in varied manners to chronic illness in others; yet most have similar emotions. Indeed, some of their reactions are probably more pronounced than in the chronically ill people they deal with.

O.K., let's begin to look at the wiggles now (or should I call them "wobbles" at lower level). Probably the best starting point is at the rock bottom level—Crashing. I have already said that this level is one to *rise from,* not *drop through.* Unfortunately though, it is one which nearly all chronically ill people *and* those who are one step away taste at least once. There is even a response to long-term illness that is quite common to Crashing. I call it

I Give Up

Yesterday's newspaper always tells the stories of many who literally passed on from this level. I have already told you as vividly as I was able about my feelings during that night in

Rochester after I was told about MS and Ronald Pruet. That was my single intense exposure to complete desolation. It was triggered by cold disclosure of what *seemed* to be truth. There are many other more common causes which bring on Crashing in people: for instance, business pressures, disappointment in love, hate, or fear. Any of these anxieties can lead an individual to I Give Up, a response too dangerous to retain.

To find out just how serious this particular response can be, ask any doctor or nurse whether the two imaginary cases that I describe now are possible or not.

The first patient has symptoms that are so radical that to every observer his battle to survive is hopeless. You can be sure too that the "hopeless" idea has occurred to him personally. The second person has an illness or wound with symptoms which do not seem nearly so serious. On the surface there is every apparent reason to expect early recovery. Yet this second patient is despondent, uncertain, and discouraged. Both patients have been exposed to I Give Up.

For the first case, as the days drag on, there is still no *physical* improvement. However for no obvious reason he begins to shake off his depressed outlook. For the second, as time passes there is no physical or mental improvement, although there should be.

The first case, now strengthened by medical treatment *and* change of soul, begins a long battle to improve. The second, supported by medical treatment which is more than counterbalanced by continued I Give Up, does not recover.

I Give Up can assume many faces. I wonder if sometimes it is even hidden to those who adopt this reaction at the Crashing level. I wonder if that second case in the hospital actually knew how important to his continued life it was for him to leave an attitude of defeat behind. I wonder what made him stop caring.

Another example is one which I decided at first *not* to explore, namely, the one who decides to end his own life. But the suicide of a successful business executive was headline news recently, and it changed my mind. His associates could find no specific reason for his jumping from his office window—no financial theft, no family problems, no failing health—only unsolved business pressures. In one short instant he decided that he could face his problems no longer. He Gave Up. To me his approach represents total defeat of a weak, selfish character. But that assessment seems to be quite unfair, according to published analyses of his family and associates.

If the views of others who knew him are correct, his death points primarily to one fact: I Give Up is a very dangerous emotion, one which can destroy in a matter of seconds the very life of a person who harbors the emotion. Avoid it.

Other statistics show that with the lower national speed limits there are fewer highway deaths. Those same statistics do not reveal, however, those highway deaths that are caused by drivers who have given up the whole game. I saw a recent discussion which suggested that many accidents are simply a means to self-destruction for drivers afflicted with I Give Up. How many? I don't know. Why? I don't know. If the idea is correct, however, we can be sure that I Give Up could even be dangerous to us as blameless drivers, as well as to several innocent highway bridges.

One final example of this approach might be the man who has suffered a chronic, confining illness which restricts both his outlook and his life style. Perhaps he was an athlete before. Or perhaps he was the manager or driving force of a large business. After the interruption he is faced with adjusting to a radical change or accepting a very short life span. If he doesn't adjust to changes, has he embraced I Give Up as his reaction? In other words, does he want an early end in much the same way as any other potential suicide? Give your own answer.

Check me out on those examples, will you? I cannot understand the ways that inner powers, these unspoken decisions such as I Give Up, generate such powerful changes. Just because I can't see them and don't understand them, however, doesn't mean that I can't accept the fact that they *are* real. I testify to their reality in this case not only from faith but also from personal experience with I Give Up. I've been there for both

the exposure as well as the change that can come after I Give
Up is abandoned.

Lines from a poem that I remember from my childhood
point the way better than more of my prose. They go like this:

> One ship drives east and another west
> With the selfsame winds that blow.
> 'Tis the set of the sails and not the gales
> Which decides the way to go.

> Like the winds of the sea
> Are the ways of fate
> As we voyage along through life.
> It's the will of the soul that decides the goal
> And not the calm or the strife.

Most of the "wiggles on the hook" come at levels higher
than Crashing. There is one response though which is probably
common to *all* the groups at *all* levels at *some time*. If you are
alive, you will recognize that you have used the wiggle I call

Why Me?

This reaction is so common because it is not necessarily tied
to health; rather it seems to be dictated by chance. For instance,
suppose that you are a student in a class of 200; you haven't
studied; the professor calls on you for an answer. What do you
ask yourself? "Why Me?" Suppose that you are driving a borrowed car without your driving license; you pass through a
speed trap, and the officer stops you. What do you ask yourself
after he sends you off? "Why Me?"

Suppose that you are living in the Southwest; the chance
for contracting a rare disease like multiple sclerosis there during
any one year is one in 200,000, maybe even 500,000; you catch
it. What do you ask yourself? "Why Me?" (At least *I* did.)

Think about two more types of "Why Me?" You are in
Vietnam during a rocket attack. A shattering blast comes. Your
best friend is killed; another friend escapes without a scratch.
Through the pain and haze you realize that you are alive, but
you see your shoe—with your foot in it across the room. Days
later you ask, "Why Me?"

You are happily married to one who has become, without

advance notice, chronically ill. Your careful plans for the future no longer apply. It is natural for you to ask, when you see routines that you enjoyed earlier continue for others without you, "Why Me?"

To some people, the reaction to illness is sharp and bitter; while others seem indifferent or even whimsical. Who knows, to a very few there may be no reaction at all.

Let me tell those of you who do not have chronic illness a fable that, as I see it, describes the response of many of those "Why Me?'s" to their situation. When it's finished, I'll explain why the fable might be a pretty good answer to the common question.

In this land of fable and imagination where we journey, your parents are Father Fate and Lady Luck, a very formidable couple, respected or feared by all. You and your sisters named Mary and Betty, and your brothers, Joe and John, have matured in comfort after lo these many years in a rural setting.

All five of you agree that your parents have two strong character traits that you can absolutely rely on: (1) Both parents are completely impartial in their attention and favor to their family of five children. In other words, there is no question in anyone's mind about one child being favored over another. (2) Both parents exercise stern control and are unyielding after they make their decisions. This means that each child has been trained to accept his particular gift, share, or lot.

You have asked Father Fate and Lady Luck the reasons why sometimes they are very generous, while at times they are very cruel. Their only explanation is that their god named Chance directs every verdict.

One day in early spring your parents called all the children together. They told you, "You are grown men and women now. As is our custom, we will leave now for Greener Fields. We may or may not be with you in the future wherever you are in the same way

*that we are with you at this moment. After we leave,
however, you will be given gifts to remember us by.*

"Children, here's what we have arranged for you.
Our god named Chance has five sons. He will send one
son to each one of you with our gift of a share of the
farm where we have been living. Chance has assured
us that all of the farm is divided between you five, but
he has not told us which one of you gets what part of
the farm." Without saying more, Father Fate and
Lady Luck left you.

The next day Kismet, the first of Chance's sons,
came to Mary as she cooked the noon meal. He told
her, "You are a lucky one. You have been given the
house and all its furnishings. Security and safety are
yours if you find the right companion."

On the following day came the second of Chance's
sons, Fortuity. He called out John and said to him,
"You get all the green fields, all the farm lands, and
the stream in the meadow. If you keep them well, fortune and happiness are yours."

Adventure, the third of Chance's sons, came riding
on a spirited white horse the next day. He called out
to Joe, "At the direction of Chance for Father Fate
and Lady Luck I give you all the horses and wild animals. Catch them if you can! With them excitement
and fame can be yours."

Then came Destiny, fourth son of Chance. He
sought out Betty and told her, "You own all the cattle,
all the farm equipment, and the big red barn. All the
hay to feed the livestock and the pens where you will
feed them during winter snows are yours too. You see,
I give you both plenty and—plenty to do."

That night you and Betty were talking. She said,
"I don't know why I got that share of the farm. Why
should I take care of cattle for the rest of my life?
Oh, mine is the unhappy lot!"

"But what about me?" you asked Betty. "I don't

know what my share will be; only that something will be mine. . . . There is still a possibility that Chance will send me hidden treasure."

Late the next day the last son of Chance came to the door. You stepped back involuntarily when you saw that he was the blind son named named Accident. All you could do when he called your name was to answer with a mixture of fear and trembling.

"Yours is the last share," he said in a low voice. "The whole farm is already divided between the others. I bring you nothing from Father Fate and Lady Luck that you want, no promises, no explanation—only a challenge. Look on the ground in the feedlot near the barn. It's yours. Make of it what you can!" And then he vanished.

Haltingly you moved out of the security of the house to the feedlot. A single animal was shifting uneasily in the shadows there—a strange looking pony with a dirty, pale coat.

The only thing on the ground was manure.

"A bitter, sarcastic fable," you say. Maybe so, but your reaction proves to me that you don't like to be in the place of that ill-fated fifth child. I confess that neither I nor any other person who is chronically ill enjoys it either.

But don't think that the bitter approach is where I want to leave you. Remember when we first started this section that I said there is probably "Why Me?" at every soul level. At Crashing one is likely to ask that question over and over. Repetition leads to bitterness and frustration when there is no apparent answer to *any* question, and "Why Me?" is no exception to the rule.

At Quiet Desperation, the "Why Me?" question still has no answer, but it does not come up so often. The *thought* of hope at this level dampens the bitterness and frustration.

The question is asked even more rarely at the Coping level. Somehow the question shifts to "How Can I Manage?"

Those who rise to Prevailing ask "Why Me?" very rarely. This is true because the world which the chronically ill live in at this level is much larger, and they deal with more people. Another way to express this is to say that they have become "outer directed" (other people directed) in contrast to the more common "inner directed" (myself directed) thinking at Crashing. We will become better acquainted with Prevailing later.

Further attempts to answer "Why Me?" are presumptive and far too general. I will venture one more opinion though, which might be of some comfort. I do not believe that anyone is *chosen* to suffer. I do not believe that if only you had been kinder to Aunt Minnie, you would not be suffering now. I cannot believe that it is God's will for most of you to be ill. The best way to answer the perplexing question, "Why Me?" is with a couple of lines from an old hymn:

We'll talk it over in the bye and bye.

I'll ask the reason; He'll tell me why.

7

Healing—Medical and Faith

Continuing to explore the ways that people react to chronic illness, let's leave the desolate plains of Crashing behind. I found nothing attractive at that level. Instead move up with me to the foothills where Hope lives. That elusive feeling called Hope is sometimes so faint that he is only a glimmer in the distance when we struggle in Quiet Desperation. Later in the rolling hills of Coping, Hope sometimes becomes so strong, so supportive that he is as real as one of our best friends. And then unpredictably after a while he becomes only a memory.

Of course I cannot describe all of the varied approaches, the diverse specific wiggles, used by those with all manners of continuing afflictions. What a horrible thought! However, people with cancer, heart trouble, arthritis, accidents and wounds, muscular dystrophy, epilepsy, MS—the list seems to go on and on—all probably have at least one reaction in common from time to time. They adopt the wiggle which I call

Find Another Doctor

Before I begin a closer look at this approach (name it F.A.D.) that we use when things don't move the way we want them to, let me introduce you to a widow who had a chronic illness. This particular woman was pretty well off financially when her female trouble began twelve years earlier. She went first to the doctor in her home town. He prescribed as best he knew—

no results. Her immediate reaction was F.A.D.; so she went to a physician who had a reputation for results in a nearby city. He prescribed a cure, charged her quite a bit more than the first doctor, but the results were just as discouraging. This same routine went on for twelve whole years as she tried both physician (F.A.D.) and fad to find a cure. In this case at least, the best medical advice in the country as well as "the latest thing" that had helped her neighbor Mary did only one thing for her—use up all her money.

We'll meet this lady again, but right now we can agree on one simple point: No matter what the illness, F.A.D. is an expensive wiggle. It takes a lot of time and can, if carried to extremes, use up every resource we have. In addition to the high cost which is involved in all chronic illness, we have something else in common. We are continually seeking, with varying degrees of urgency, the best medical advice available. Most of us would dedicate all that we could muster in money, time, and effort to regaining the level of physical friskiness that we enjoyed long ago—so long ago that it is only a dim memory.

I started with medical advice in my search for that common gift that most do not appreciate until they lose it—health. A definition of the word *doctor* is simply "one who is trained in and licensed to practice medicine." What more logical place to begin than with the advice from one skilled in the practice of the medical arts? Why then didn't I stop after I received my first advice? My answer to that one is the same as most who suffer from a lingering illness: I kept looking for what I hadn't received yet, a complete cure.

It is probably important to separate the doctors who are *licensed* to practice medicine, the M.D.'s, from other practitioners—"doctors" who may be either self-trained or skilled in other methods of treating symptoms and are *not* recognized by licensed physicians. I distinguish between the two by changing the capitalization of Find Another Doctor, F.A.D., to lower case f.a.d., find another director.

"Wait a minute! That doesn't really show the difference in

the training and scientific approach of licensed physicians from those others who might even be frauds!" I hear some of you protest.

Quite simply I say, "Show me results that I want—that complete cure—and I'll take it no matter whom it comes from!"

Yes, you are right. Anyone who wants something like health *can* be flimflammed. I certainly don't recommend paying for promises that can't be delivered, but I want the option to look at all promised help, and then to make up my own mind. I've tried a variety of licensed physicians and specialists as well as a few unlicensed ideas. To date none of them has shown me the way to recover the level of physical health and activity that I had before 1963. What's more, the course of MS is such that it gave me a wheelchair as a present last Christmas. Do you blame me for trying both F.A.D. and f.a.d.?

Let me share with you my personal encounters with F.A.D. My purpose is not to impress you with numbers or variety; rather it is to show the driving force that I know is common in the chronically ill to regain health as long as there is hope. I began the reaction in Midland with my general practitioner, a doctor who is licensed but does not specialize. As you might guess, he was sympathetic about symptoms but not very helpful in diagnosing what was the matter. He recommended my first specialist in F.A.D., a urologist, a doctor who deals with the genitourinary tract. Results negative.

F.A.D. led me to seek my second specialist in short order, this time an internal medicine specialist, a doctor that specializes in diagnosing and treating nonsurgical diseases. Little did I know that after my problem was diagnosed that specialists would become routine. Results this time, however, again inconclusive. F.A.D.

Almost simultaneous to seeing my first two specialists a peculiar symptom involving my sight developed. This problem led me to an ophthalmologist, a physician who treats diseases of the eye. His help was similar to the other doctors that had advised me—supportive but not corrective.

A short time later, at the suggestion of my G.P., I sought the advice from a neurologist, a physician skilled in the diagnosis and treatment of the nervous system. All of this variety of specialists came before the internist even suggested that I might have to go to the hospital for a better disagnosis. F.A.D.

O.K. now, let's hurry this long list along and bring it up to date, because after I started the hospital approach I seemed to multiply the number of specialists instead of adding them one by one. During that first hospital stay I added one more internist and a neurologist in Abilene and then at least three more neurologists in the Mayo Clinic. When I lived in Austin, I added one more G.P. and another internist to the list. In Oxford I have used another local G.P. as well as an internist and a neurologist in Memphis.

It is amazing to me—and a little frightening—to total the number of licensed physicians that I have seen during this long bout with MS. I have sought advice and treatment from at least three general practitioners, one ophthalmologists, a urologist, four internal medicine specialists, and seven neurologists. That adds up to a minimum of sixteen doctors that I have consulted *more* than once each. I don't intend to imply that I have used that many doctors at once, but rather that I have regularly become dissatisfied with comparing the results gained to the results hoped for. I realize that over a long period with one illness that many others have seen more doctors, suffered more, and spent more. All I am trying to point out is simply this: One common wiggle sought again and again was Find Another Doctor.

To those of us not satisfied with the results of F.A.D. there is always the alternative of f.a.d., those innovations which physicians sometimes tolerate, sometimes deplore. I hesitate to list the whole range of different approaches I have considered. If I did, it might seem that all I do—night and day—is to look inward selfishly. Those of you without daily, sometimes constant, reminders of infirmity cannot understand. Those who have them will. Actually, most of us who have a long history of F.A.D. probably entertain f.a.d. alternatives without admitting to ourselves that we are only entertaining an important guest, Hope.

One f.a.d. move which I tried for about six months not so long ago was inspired by a picture of an elderly man in a national newspaper. The picture showed this happy man who, according to his claim, had completely recovered from MS, as shown by his balancing on one leg and smiling happily. His cure of the until then incurable MS was developed by his own use of a diet with no gluten. (I don't know what it is, but it sounds like we *should* do without it.) The information which he freely sent on my inquiry described his diet in detail: no cereals, low fat, no sugar, supplemented only by vitamins. I could see no harm in that approach. Even my neurologist could see no harm; but, of course, he scoffed at the possibility of favorable results. You know, I was faithful to that diet for a while, but I lacked the patience to continue as long as the man recommended. Could this have been a personal cure that I abandoned too soon? Whether it was or not, I will probably never know because "logic" convinced me that it was a slim chance.

Another f.a.d. tack that I was sorely tempted to try was the use of mega-doses (very large numbers) of vitamins. Logic supported the chance that in my body there was an imbalance of the vital minerals. Too, the one recommending this approach was a licensed physician. He even sent the recommended formula for taking the pills and injections. Furthermore, his general idea was supported by a distinguished professor whom I met at Texas University. The idea was shelved because of unfavorable publicity in recent medical publications and by the fact that I could not get a local doctor to assist in the injections recommended in this approach. Besides, my "patience supply" had already been found to be too low for promises without quick change.

Chiropractors claim to have cured or at least lightened the load of MS. I tried that approach only once, admittedly not enough for results. Perhaps with endurance on my part they could help, but chances for a real change through a chiropractor are not appealing.

Still another f.a.d. that I have considered but not tried is the use of acupuncture, the Chinese treatment for many ills. I would happily endure needles stuck in the prescribed skilled manner *if* I could have quick results. None has been promised, and I have not tried acupuncture.

The grapevine which transmits information about f.a.d. is fed by unsupported rumor as well as results reported from fellow sufferers. The chronically ill person who plays the f.a.d. game from Quiet Desperation has an entirely different attitude from those who are more stable in Coping or Prevailing. For instance, I understand "from reliable sources" that a new medicine which successfully treats MS has been discovered in Russia (or was it China?). There is a doctor in a small Mississippi town near Oxford who has treated MS with spinal injections. As a result, one man recovered full mobility from earlier confinement in a wheelchair. All these are probably great examples of f.a.d., but I have no desire to trace them out.

The possibilities of f.a.d., no matter what the disease, are almost endless. Most of those chances, however, are quite a bit more expensive than a ticket to the Irish Sweepstakes, and unfortunately, offer just about the same chances for a health "fortune."

Let's return now to that woman you met a little bit ago—you know, the one with the female trouble that spent all her money on F.A.D. Instead of feeling better, at the end of twelve years she was actually quite a bit worse. You can sympathize with the mounting feeling of desperation that she probably felt as she worried about her future—without health or wealth.

Then she heard about a traveling preacher. The stories that she heard around some of the shops downtown were that He was truly a miracle worker. Why Sarah told of actually seeing old crippled George walking again, and of blind Jim claiming to see now—both after their meeting this strange preacher!

She probably argued with her "better judgment" like this: "I've tried the best that doctors can tell me, but nothing has happened. I'm getting so weak now that I can't do what I need to do around the house. But, really now, how could I possibly go up to a stranger and ask for a miracle? How could I say to a *man* who is not a doctor .that I've got this trouble. that women sometimes have and it won't go away—so please heal it? How ridiculous! Besides, what if He asked for money?" I rather expect that the argument went on for weeks.

She finally resolved her inner argument this way: "I know what—I won't even talk to Him personally. I hear that large crowds follow Him around. What I'll do is just mingle with the people that are close to Him. If He really is what they say He is—a miracle worker—just *touching* Him might give me that miracle that I want. He wouldn't even have to know."

Many of you recognize the woman's story now. She got her miracle because the traveling preacher was Jesus. The time that this took place was nearly two thousand years ago. You see, we haven't changed much as the years pass by. The problems which we all face are pretty much the same. I am convinced too that the emotions that go with chronic illness are not much different. Just as that woman did, so do many of us react by seeking a religious solution to our problems with a wiggle I call

God Can Heal

I feel uncertain, maybe even defensive, about what you are thinking now that I have introduced "faith healing" as a possible reaction, a wiggle, for chronic illness. Those of you who remember what I've already said—that I am a Christian and that I have experienced answers to prayer—have probably "locked in" an impression of what's coming. One group will expect, almost automatically, a formula whereby all chronically ill people can regain complete health, or *Conquering,* if only they would follow the steps: No. 1, No. 2, and thus, No. 3. Sorry to disappoint you, but I won't even pretend to suggest that.

Others might skip quickly over any words which even mention God, Christ, and healing. After all, I have told you that I'm not a preacher and do not claim to be an authority. Slow down a little, though; I have a few interesting ideas to share.

Still others will remember that long list of F.A.D. and f.a.d. reactions and then reasonably ask, "If faith healing is available in this age, why aren't you well now?"

That is another of your questions that really challenges me. In order to answer that question, I intend to show you what I learned about faith healing. I am reasonably certain that you will not be satisfied at my approach or my answer. For that matter, neither am I. The full answer to that question will probably be explained and understood at the same time I know "Why Me?"

The closest I had ever been to faith healing in my life was reading about examples in the Bible. As a kid, I had heard about but never seen mysterious meetings way out "in the country." (Now that's false superiority if I ever heard of it, since I lived in a "city" of about six thousand people.) At these meetings of what we called Holy Rollers, some supposedly spoke "in tongues" (languages that nobody understood), and there might have been "laying on of hands" to heal sickness. I was not curious enough to find out then, and until about four years ago I had never seen it tried. Furthermore, as a well-educated, reasonably well-balanced man, I had not considered faith healing to be even a legitimate wiggle.

One day I responded to a persistent invitation from friends who knew about MS and me to come to a meeting of a small prayer group in Oxford. There was no shouting, no "rolling" but there was praise and a feeling of peace. I was impressed. In a similar meeting the next week the same pattern was followed: songs, prayers, praise, and then requests for special prayer. I asked, with some hesitation, for prayer to improve my health—to Conquer MS—in the same manner that the group used before for other individuals with other illnesses. In a matter of minutes these dedicated individuals were "laying hands" on my head, praying for my healing. I remembered the promise when Christ said that all things are possible if only His disciples ask, believing that it is done.

We asked, believing, but Ronald Pruet still had MS when we finished. What did I think? Wasn't it discouraging?

My impressions of this encounter with faith healing corresponded to my earlier belief in God. You see, *my* God is the Creator, He is all-powerful, eternal, and all-knowing; yet He loves and cares for individuals. Obviously, one such as He *can* heal. He did heal all kinds of disease ages ago; so all I had to do was find what He requires to do it now.

Seeking an answer, I attended other prayer groups. After all, others might have a more direct channel. I studied the Bible more diligently, since it is His Word. I prayed regularly. All of this was probably well and good in itself; yet something about it all didn't seem quite right. I had been told by some that my purpose should be praise—not healing. Others said I should seek "deliverance" from demons, an idea that I could not seriously entertain. Others said that I should become more dedicated, and thus worthier of God's healing. But I could not find in the Bible where Christ made the ones that He healed to become worthy of or qualified for His blessing.

Go back to that woman with the female trouble again. When she approached Christ in the crowd, touched His robe, and then was healed, do you imagine that she came to Him with anything else on her mind except that she might be healed? Do you think that she praised Him *first* and *then* touched the robe? It certainly seems logical to me that she wanted to be healed of a twelve-year-old illness over all possible goals, and her main qualification was simply to seek Him.

I wasn't satisfied with the healing answers that I had received and was intrigued by the phenomenal reports about the ministry of Kathryn Kuhlman. Too, I had heard of similar results that often happened when Oral Roberts preached. Because of the possibility that results would come more readily in a mass meeting, I decided to go when I heard about a Kathryn Kuhlman service that was coming soon in Monroe, Louisiana. Myra Sue and I drove to Cajun country.

About mid-afternoon before the scheduled night meeting, the lobby of the Civic Auditorium began to fill and then was soon jammed to capacity. Small groups, most of whom had come from nearby communities, sang hymns, prayed, and simply "visited." All denominations were present, and everyone shared in a flood of emotions that ranged all the way from skepticism to absolute certainty that miracles were minutes away.

The service began with spirited singing of hopeful hymns. At the right moment Kathryn Kuhlman swept onto the elevated stage, dressed in a long white gown which reflected the spotlights. I could tell that her showmanship was polished, smoothed by carefully synchronized timing and repetition. Yet her announced purpose was only to witness about Christ and the Holy Spirit. She was careful to give Them all the glory. Nothing that *she* did could heal anyone. That fact was the substance of her simple message to the packed hall that night.

Then she testified that healing had occurred for those afflicted with a specific disease, first one illness and then another. At the same time she asked that those who experienced healing to identify themselves and come forward. Hands were raised in different sections of the congregation of about three thousand people, and as the service continued there must have been almost two hundred who came to the stage. They told their backgrounds—some educated and some not, some black and some white, some old and some very young. After each told of his miracle, Miss Kuhlman touched him on the head. An amazing thing then happened—the person who was healed was so stunned that he slumped to the floor. They were, to use the figure of speech commonly used to describe the phenomenon, "slain in the Spirit." It happened so regularly that men who assist Miss Kuhlman were prepared each time to catch the people before they fell.

I spoke to one who testified publicly that she had been healed of MS in an earlier meeting in Tulsa. She had come to Monroe only to share her experience. When I asked her how I could receive the same blessing she said, "Only believe."

When the meeting ended I had not received that special "tingling" that signified a healing experience. I believed as strongly as I was able, but all that I could truthfully say that

I received was a good workout from a trying day. I had trouble walking before the meeting—I probably had a little more difficulty after it was over. Was it my fault? Was it Miss Kuhlman's fault? Was it God's fault?

That night in the motel I asked myself those three questions. Whatever the answers, the actual results of the meeting were too painful to discuss with Myra Sue. The hope that had caused me to come to Monroe was tested, had been found wanting, and was replaced by the commonplace planning for my coming week as a professor at Ole Miss.

You know, that Kuhlman service was probably the high point of my exposure to faith healing as a legitimate reaction to chronic illness. Since then the intensity of seeking deliverance or healing has lessened. Oh, don't get me wrong. I know that God can heal; it's just that I don't feel the fervor, the urgency to seek it that I did then. It may be that His implied direction to *wait* is really the only answer He intends.

I notice this change too: During the last couple of years, my desire to participate in fervent prayer groups has gone down. It may be my imagination, but I feel that likewise the groups are glad to see one of their unanswered prayer problems wander away.

"Wait a minute!" I can almost hear you say. "You've told us of a few experiences with faith healing but you never did say what you actually thought about it."

I do believe that you are either less hesitant to pin me down as we become better acquainted or that you just want a direct answer to a tough question that puzzles you too.

So then, just how does faith healing fit in for you and me today? Let's look first at the source and then at how it comes.

The source of *all* healing for *all* diseases, I've been told by physicians, is a matter of question. Some give nature the credit; some medicine; some the will; some God; but all use the training and experience that has produced healing for them before. We could agree that *faith* healing, defined as healing without medicine, comes from God. Now everyone probably has his own picture of God, but I refer you in this case to the definition of *my* God that I've already told you about.

Now the second question, *how* can faith healing become a reality instead of a promise? As a result of mass meetings directed by famous healers? After prayer from small dedicated groups? Only after study, prayer, and praise? With fasting (going without food and drink)? Let's explore some answers.

I've read books and pamphlets by dedicated ministers who give specific "how to" directions. Most of these preachers reveal directions from the Holy Spirit since they are, after all, "charismatic." That's religious language that means baptized in the Spirit and gifted with "speaking in unknown tongues." I don't criticize them for being charismatic because I too was "baptized in the Holy Spirit" (though I never could speak in tongues). What I strongly disagree with in many of their verbal and written opinions is when they imply, sometimes even promise, that healing will come after certain steps are followed faithfully.

Now, just a minute! We are supposedly praying to the same God. God as I picture Him, however, cannot be bundled into a neat package and then unwrapped at our convenience for healing. In the case of specifying the steps for one who is ill to climb for healing, I think that any organized pattern is at its best missing the mark, and at its worse a cruel deception.

Then at the other extreme view, books have been published which "prove" that healing miracles do not actually take place today. For example, in the Kuhlman services or the Oral Roberts meetings, exercises in mob psychology produce temporary changes in selected subjects who are suffering from psychosomatic illness. "Careful" documentation shows that no real healing miracles take place in those meetings.

Hogwash!

Excuse me, but the one word reaction tells just how I feel. A more polite reply would be this: Authors who feel called on to disprove modern faith healing commit what economists and students of logic call a "fallacy of composition." This means that their reasoning leads them to make general conclusions from limited data. In other words, they infer that because of exceptions that they have ferreted out about the reality of claimed faith healing, there is no faith healing at all today. Personal observation and experience convince me that they too miss the mark.

What do I personally think about faith healing then? Frankly, I believe in its *reality* after exploring the idea for over four years. Just as I have indicated, however, I do not believe that I can summon the healing I need; nor do I think that I can earn it. As I see it, the whole thing comes down to a question of grace—an unmerited gift—from the Supplier.

Paul talks in one of his letters about God, the source of faith healing. He pointed out that just as God had told Moses earlier, God has mercy on whom He pleases to have mercy on. Likewise, He will show compassion (I'll call it healing) on whomever He chooses. Then Paul goes on to point out that God did, after all, control our own creation.

Speaking to those of us who might question the fairness of His choices, Paul added, "Who are you to criticize your Maker? Does the clay criticize the Potter who shaped it?"

I couldn't answer those questions in a way that satisfied me. I thought about those passages in the Bible quite a bit more though. Somehow the very questions themselves resolved the dilemma. When I accepted the Potter-clay or Father-son relationship for God and me, a strange new peace came to my soul.

8

Reactions at Prevailing

It is easy to argue that, short of Conquering, the soul measure that I have named *Prevailing* is preferred over all others. At this level one overcomes and contributes even as the battle continues. Unfortunately though, working up to that stage *and then staying there* are not tasks that are "easy automatics" for a person with any kind of chronic illness. I have already talked about several common reactions that many of us have as we scramble up that mountain called Prevailing. Now is the time to deal with common responses that we use—either by instinct or our plan—to stay there.

Let's get at it by considering three "shades" or variations of stability (the ability to stick to it) in Prevailing. In contrast to such wiggles as "I Give Up" or "Why Me?", which usually reflect soul levels *lower* than Prevailing, all three of these reactions are usually found at the higher level. Those who use them have already scrambled up. In other words, when using these responses, those who are *struggling* with chronic illness symptoms are probably *overcoming*. The point that I intend to make is simply this: While all three responses may touch Prevailing, only *one* of these shades offers a sound approach to long-run stability. I for one have tried variations of all three. By using the preferred "shade" I intend to Prevail for a long time.

Here's a little more background as I see it. I believe that nearly everyone who is chronically ill may convince himself that he has overcome his long-term problem or is on the verge of doing so. When this happens he may have pulled himself up to Prevailing almost by his own boot straps. He may have been bolstered by a natural remission. He may have seen a friend or acquaintance with similar problem Conquer the chronic illness. Whatever the self-induced cause, he has moved past the lower levels to Prevailing.

Others may have benefited from expert medical treatment, successful physical therapy, or answered prayer. These people who have gained from the contributions of others—chronically ill though they might still be—have an improved outlook and confidence. They too have reached the level of Prevailing.

Now here's the common problem: Whatever worked to boost anyone to Prevailing may, over time, become less supportive. Most of us tend to be patient for only so long when we don't get quick results. It is human nature to cast around for another way ("F.A.D." for example) for more strength or speedier solutions. In doing so we just *might* slip off the Prevailing level.

Now that we have a better view of the main problem at Prevailing, those three "shades" of stability will have more meaning. It's not that they are unique to my experience. As a matter of fact, I am confident that you or someone you know has gone through the same responses. As we consider them together though, we both could benefit—me for organizing my thoughts, you for identifying and perhaps avoiding similar mistakes.

Almost as soon as I returned to Midland from the hospital in Abilene, my spirits soared and my outlook quickly changed from "I've been sick" to "Look out, world—here I come!" It is remarkable how my confidence grew along with my ability to function physically. Don't misunderstand—I did not switch from a protected hospital routine to the demanding business world without any difficulty. Somehow it became not so much how well I made the change; instead my confidence mushroomed according to how well I *thought* I was doing. Really, that's what confidence is, isn't it?

"So what's the matter with thinking like that?" you ask. There is absolutely nothing the matter with that kind of thinking—let's call it self-confidence. Without it there can be no success in any competitive field. Think about some of the complications that might come up, however, if self-confidence turns into pride. It is not very hard to imagine how self-confidence could even lead on the one hand to hypocrisy (pretending to be something you are not) or on the other hand to self-delusion (kidding yourself about what's real). I suspect that most of us who have been saddled with a chronic illness are acquainted with some of those complications, regardless of whether or not we recognize it.

I rather expect that ideas like these were companions to my confidence in one response in Prevailing. Even though it had been only weeks since I had been in the hospital, I convinced myself that chronic illness was *behind* me. I was quick to repeat —mentally and in conversations about MS—the phrase that labeled my Prevailing reaction then:

Ignore It.

Another name for this wiggle might be "I'm As Good As I Ever Was," or even "Yeah, I Used to Have That!" Perhaps the repeated assurance of victory when at *Coping* is enough, but in *Prevailing* it should involve more than just ignoring the chronic illness. After all, let's be realistic; how can anyone honestly overlook a symptom that hurts, that might kill him, or that affects the way he sees and walks? Maybe you can if you are a tried-and-true stoic (a person indifferent to pain), but there are not very many of you around now. Unless you flaunt illness and enjoy sympathy, it's more likely that you will mask your feelings and, depending on the circumstances, hide your health history by saying to an inquiring friend or acquaintance, "Ignore It!"

When I got back into the swing of business activity, I was anxious to show my business associates, particularly my partners, that there were no lasting effects from MS. It would be pretty accurate to say that I moved quickly from *Coping* to *Prevailing* because of the well-remembered "buy-me-out" spur that my partners had given me. Faster than my wife approved, I returned to a full work schedule, complete with assurances to all concerned that I was quite capable of anything required in my "prehospital" role. Even though I became tired much earlier than before, I was still able to do all that was needed. It didn't take long for me to convince Ronald Pruet that he was "overcoming" in fine fashion.

But there were a few unbalancing effects. For instance, the way that other people saw me then was quite important. To me it's amazing when I think about the change of attitude that developed in so short a time. In the hospital, "my" place because I had been there for nearly three months, I didn't even pause to wonder what visitors thought when they saw me stumble. But at home in Midland, actually much more "my" place since I had lived there for six years, I was horrified at the thought of making a spectacle of myself.

Think about that for a minute. Doesn't something in that reaction strike you as odd or off-key?

"Not really," you might say. "No one wants to be embarrassed."

Think again though. Doesn't my reaction imply that I thought people were basically cruel and insensitive? Shouldn't I have had enough confidence (call it self-assurance) not to care what strangers thought and faith enough to know that friends and family understand?

I didn't stop at trying to hide all effects of my illness. I avoided exposure to anyone else who was afflicted with MS. I feel sure, in view of the fact that I was then mobile and blessed with full sight, hearing, and clear speech, that I didn't want to *see* the full range of possible symptoms of MS. I remember one man in Midland who had MS. He walked with a cane and was active in the National Multiple Sclerosis Society. I saw him occasionally, but I didn't pursue common interests. Perhaps I didn't have the courage to walk in his shoes.

You know, when I reminisce about that period when I *thought* I was *Prevailing*, I find that I just might have been *hiding*. When pride told me how well I was doing, I listened. It turned out, however, that my acquaintance who had MS was reacting in a manner which was stronger and much more beneficial to others. My deep-seated reaction then was inner directed, full of doubt and uncertainty. My mask to society was, of course, just the opposite. It was only later that I realized that there was little depth and sustaining strength in my reaction that was grounded in pride and deception.

I don't remember what triggered my feeling of dissatisfaction at "Ignore It." Perhaps it was guilt at seeing others admit physical suffering while I tried to hide any effects of mine. Perhaps I was afraid of the predicted course of MS. Perhaps one cannot be truly satisfied with his life if he is not on a course that he charts as true. Whatever the cause, I decided that *Prevailing* by blandly saying "Ignore It" to my associates as well as to myself was not good enough. I liked the level where I was; but I made up my mind to find an honest, more open way to stay there.

I was very fortunate to have a job waiting when I came back to Midland, one to which I happily gave both my interest and time. Added to that was a circle of friends and a place òr two in monthly bridge clubs for friend wife and me. What's more, there was always a church meeting on nearly any night of the week. Given these sources of business, social, and religious activity, it was easy for me to make a smooth transition to another shade of Prevailing stability, one which I call

Stay Busy

One of the most important requirements for anyone who Prevails is an absorbing, challenging, demanding channel for his daily interests. It seems to me that the actual activity could vary all over the map because people are not the same, and chronic illnesses are different. Creative art might fill the bill for one, while earning a livelihood would be what another needs. In my case the need to earn a living for my family was a pressing requirement that I felt quite strongly when I returned to Midland. For truly, *at the time* it was what I needed to Prevail. I was very busy.

One encouraging development in our society is the recognition in government and industry that the chronically ill or handicapped need that absorbing channel I speak of. Furthermore, there is recognition—much broader than many handicapped are aware of—that handicapped workers *can* find a meaningful slot in the work force. "Vocational Rehabilitation" is the name for the type of training which balances what the handicapped lacks with what he is capable of doing. The proficiency levels that may be reached by hard work, determination, and training are astounding. It goes without saying that those who reach these levels have overcome and thus *Prevail*. At the same time, they have shifted from the role of "Receiver" to "Contributor." Let me stress that it is not so much the amount they contribute but the fact that they know they don't always receive without giving something.

I have described how my pressing requirement shifted in about two years from earning the daily bread as a leasing company manager to learning the daily lessons as a graduate student. I realize that I was very fortunate to have that opportunity. But you know, more education is not out of the reach of anyone today, regardless of his health. For example, there are night courses in colleges, correspondence courses that could be prepared at home, as well as enrollment as a regular student in colleges and universities. Perhaps I am more tuned to it than most, but it seems to me that the handicapped are more and more common on today's campuses. No one is given a grade he doesn't earn in the circles where I move. All participants gain, no matter what the grade, by stimulating their souls.

Actually, as I talk about the reaction I call "Stay Busy," it seems to me that two of the more productive and satisfying ways of playing the game are the pursuit of a meaningful occupation and training the "thinking part" that we all have. None of us ever reaches a level of learning with no more ignorance to instruct. In today's economy it is a rare person who does not need just a bit more income too.

But "Stay Busy" as a reaction in Prevailing may involve many different outlets, some of which may not be so productive. Indeed some outlets probably satisfy only a frightened need for scheduling every minute of every day. When this complication to the reaction develops, satisfaction—sometimes more than Prevailing—becomes a goal instead of a feeling.

For instance, have you ever scheduled a frantic flurry of activity that really does nothing more than blot out idle thoughts, instead of becoming that absorbing interest that we all need? Check me out on this opinion of mine, will you: A moderate amount of the following activities is helpful; too much becomes an unproductive escape.

How about daily games of bridge?

How about TV day and night?

How about daily worries about tomorrow?

How about monitoring your own illness daily? hourly?

How about becoming identified as one with your particular kind of chronic illness instead of as a real person who, by the way, is ill?

How about searching for the latest medical, fad, or faith wiggles?

I can hear some of you snort and then say, "You've stopped talking and have started meddling!"

As I looked more closely at "Stay Busy," I was struck by the fact that the actual overall needs of anyone Prevailing are really not different from the long-run needs of any healthy person. When "Stay Busy" does *not* provide a balanced, outward-looking approach, it may shorten our stay at the higher soul level.

You know, all of this talk about Prevailing, handicaps, wiggles, reactions—you name it—shows me something that just might be important to anyone with a chronic illness or a handicap. What we need is a response to our problems that will not only keep us at the soul level that we want but also serve us when we progress even further to complete recovery. This thought leads me to the last and *best* wiggle, which I have named

Accept—Adjust—Amend

I could easily name this response the "Triple A Approach," or some other catchy phrase; but a "cute" name might tend to downgrade its importance. Let me enlarge on the meaning of each of the three action verbs—*Accept, Adjust, Amend*—that make up the name. It is appropriate that you recognize that each word in the three-part name calls for action, sometimes even change. Still more important than the implied action, I suggest that this particular response to chronic troubles should lead to greater stability.

Beginning with the word *Accept*, picture two meanings of "accepting" to one who is chronically ill. The word *Accept* has many definitions in daily use, but in this wiggle the meanings which I draw on are "to take with good grace" and "to acknowledge as received." As I see it, both meanings are important to this response.

One who is chronically ill usually must be helped *at some stage*—in the hospital, at home, at work—*at some time*. Accepting help when we can't help ourselves is almost automatic. Accepting help when we can do it ourselves could be habit forming. Taking the right amount with good grace is a problem which only the individual can solve, for his own case.

But really that part of "accepting" is not the major problem for most chronically ill people. One of the hardest things to admit to ourselves is that we just might not be as good as we ever were. In the response labeled "Ignore It" I talked about the time when I "rose above" MS by refusing to accept the fact that I had the disease. For a short period I was able to fool myself—and maybe most others too. For the long run though, the game got too tiresome to continue.

I finally accepted the fact that something had happened; my planned life style was interrupted. But get this point straight: *The only thing I needed to "acknowledge as received" was the fact that a change had come about.* I did not need to accept the "way things were" because I had been sick. *Status quo I could change.*

All of this brings me to the second and probably the most

important word of Accept—Adjust—Amend. One important definition of the word *Adjust* is "to bring the parts of anything to a true or more effective relative position." A second common meaning is "to offset an error." Both of these definitions are vital parts of this reaction. I'll deal with both of them.

You will remember that I said that we all had three parts in common: body, soul, and spirit. It is significant to realize that in the case of chronic illness one or more of our three "parts" is out of its "true and effective relative position." The *reason* for the problem is basic to its correction, but for the purpose of this response it is secondary to accepting the fact that something is "out of kilter" or "out of true" *and* that it needs adjusting.

I think that *balance* is an absolute requirement to a stable approach to the daily demands of our life. By balance I mean a mixture of body (the physical), soul (mind, emotions, mental), and spirit (spiritual), which when properly combined offers a blended response to problems. Unadjusted chronic illness makes balance impossible.

"Too fuzzy," you say.

All right, how about this? A phrase that is commonly used by young people is "Put it all together now." What I suggest is simply this: When part of you hurts, or your soul is torn apart, or your spirit is looking for answers that aren't there, you cannot put it all together. Adjustments have to be made.

What you or I need from time to time is this adjustment exercise:

1. Stop what we are doing.
2. Assess (gauge, measure, look at) where we are.
3. Find out what we want.
4. Measure what we need to get it.
5. Adjust physically and mentally as much as possible to reach the goals.

"Aw," you ask me, "what good will a general approach like that do for *my* problem?"

Unquestionably, those generalities won't solve anything. But when you give specific answers—more specific than blue sky, mother, and apple pie answers—something can happen. If you can't decide yourself what the answers to your special need or needs are, you need help. Ask for it.

What I am getting at in all of this is that each of us must recognize what is the "weakest part" or the part that is out of its *effective relative position*.

When we find it (and we know that the culprit may change from one period to another), we are ready for the second meaning of the word *Adjust*, namely, "to offset an error." Just as before, the reason for the error is secondary. Offsetting it to gain greater balance is much more important. Another way to think of this correction is to "compensate" for or "counterbalance" what is lacking. If a deficiency is properly counterbalanced, the weakness is effectively replaced and its function is fulfilled.

The needed adjustment, the offsetting of an error, the counterbalancing effect—call it what you may—applies to whatever part is out of kilter—be it body, soul, or spirit. I have talked about different wiggles that many of us try for the adjustment of one or more of our three common parts. One of the main things we gain in these various reactions is satisfaction that we are doing our best to correct a weakness. Indeed, "doing our best" can become a reaction in itself, as shown in my earlier discussion of "Stay Busy."

Once we have had a meaningful, personal encounter with the first two parts of Accept—Adjust—Amend, the third segment, Amend, follows in perfect order. *Amend* as used in this reaction means "to improve or to put right." The concept of Amending blends smoothly with the idea of correcting a weakness, offsetting an error, and bringing all the parts into a more effective relative position.

As a matter of fact, the major reason for adding the word at all is emphasis on the need for *commitment to improvement*. Most of us share the common failing of putting off to the future the corrections we needed yesterday. We may go through the steps of accepting the problem, deciding on adjustments needed, and then simply postpone the whole thing until another time. Commitment to corrective action always comes before the desired change itself.

There it is then, the best explanation of Accept—Adjust—Amend that I can supply. This response to chronic illness seems to me the most productive, long lasting, flexible reaction anyone can have. It offers the "shade" of stability in Prevailing that I use now and plan to use in the future. I can look back to the way I used this reaction in the hospital in Abilene, in Rochester, in changing occupations, and in problems that I had yesterday.

Believe me, the approach as I outlined it combines reactions that I have been through. There is no reason for me to claim that it is the only way to combat problems of chronic illness. After all, just look at the different wiggles I described in the last several pages. Any one of them might be the answer for your case. I know very well that we are all different, and most of us are saddled with a different problem. The only thing I am sure of is the fact that Accept—Adjust—Amend worked the best for me.

And do you know how I know it's true? Most of the time (question the man who says *always*) I have peace. That peace is best likened to confidence, maybe even self-assurance, that I am on the right path. It might even be a taste or just a glimmer of the kind of peace Jesus was talking about when He promised a deeper peace than the world could give. Is that so strange since He is my Guide?

9

Strategy versus Tactics

Well, we've just about made it to the finish line of that whirlwind, "unaverage" journey I promised you a long way back. We drove from the west Texas plains, rushed through two hospitals, made a switch from the business world through four years of graduate school (rah, rah, Pardner) to a new occupation of college professor (one chorus of "Dixie," Suh).

Along the way we became well acquainted with my analysis of the three "people parts" that all of us have in common and my five-level Soul Scale, a scheme to compare "where you are". in chronic illness to "where you want to be."

Then I discussed eight reactions to lingering illness that many of us have tried. The wiggles that I talked about were I Give Up, Why Me?, Find Another Doctor, Find Another Director, God Can Heal, Ignore It, Stay Busy, and Accept-Adjust-Amend.

All I can say in summary is, "That was a tremendous lot of conversation!"

As I reflect on all those very personal ideas and experiences I shared, I am amazed. Quite frankly, I don't usually enjoy talking about myself—believe it or not! Candidly, in our travels together you have learned more about me, my problems, and my emotions than any other close friend that I have.

After all our twists and turns there is still one more loose end that needs to be tied up. I remember well when you asked this question: "If I want to move from one soul level to another and then hold my position in a higher stage, how can I do it?"

I really wasn't ignoring you when you asked that. It's just that your questions have gotten a lot tougher. The main thing I had to avoid was a platitude instead of a "for real" answer. You know what I mean—*not* an answer like

"Be kind to others," or

"Pray and praise three times a day," or

"Think of yourself as being well."

The in-depth answer to your question more or less distills all of my reactions to chronic illness from before I knew what it was to now. And I hope I haven't stopped learning.

You have seen of course that moving *down* the Soul Scale is no problem at all. All that anyone has to do is relax, feel very sorry for himself, and in no time at all he can slide from Prevailing to Crashing. But what's to be gained from that?

It's moving *up* the scale and then holding that is the trick!

Before we go deeper in exploring the How answer, agree with me on three ground rules:

First, assume that we are on the same level now. We begin at Prevailing. Furthermore, we both have problems.

Second, as I list specific problems that I have today, you do the same thing with your own difficulties—preferably on a sheet of paper.

Third, I will outline how I seek solutions to those specific problems. Let me emphasize, I do not hold myself up to you as an example! While I tell what has been helpful to me, at no time does it mean "Do as I do."

Now here's the way we can approach your very probing question. Let's move in parallel directions—you with your problems and me with mine. When I tell you about how I attack distinct daily problems, you decide if any light has been shed on how you can defeat your difficulties.

Right now there are at least three very real problems that

confront me. (Don't let me get ahead of you. Now is the time
to list *your own* problems.)

First, I still have my very own Pale Pony—multiple sclerosis.
MS was never a frolicsome "pet" that I wanted as a companion.
As a matter of fact, during the past few years it has become
much more demanding. Three years ago, a foot brace. Two years
ago, a cane. Last year, a wheelchair. One never needs to remind me of its presence.

The second hindrance is a recurring battle with impatience,
the arch enemy to peace of mind. Impatience at the unwanted
changes in mobility. Impatience at the negative rate of physical
improvement recently.

A third major stumbling block is my lack of recognition—
you could even call it a periodic lack of trust—in the divine
plan and promise for my life. It's a classic case of "now I see
it" and "now I don't."

About 3:00 A.M. one night an idea concerning those three
difficulties became very clear to me. Each of my three people
parts is under stress from a separate problem: Body from multiple sclerosis, Soul from impatience, and Spirit from lack of
trust. In other words, I am being attacked on three fronts.

To prevent slipping downward from Prevailing, all of the
resources available must be marshalled. For Body, I should seek
the best medical advice available. (Check! I have.) For Soul,
I should focus on the love and support I have from others instead of feeling isolated. (Check! I do.) For Spirit, I should
simply rest in His hands. (Check! I try.)

"Well," you say, "if you do those things, what else is there?"

The answer to that question is closely intertwined with the
answer to your original question about how to move from one
level to another. Notice, I have said that *all* of the resources
must be gathered. Surely you don't think there's little left *of me*
to do anything *for me* in that three-front battle.

Just because you and I have had a serious interruption in
our life plan, we haven't earned the privilege of always being
cared for by others—doctors, family, and God—without any
effort from us in return. Quite the contrary—after a while it

seems to me that being coddled like that becomes a *sentence* instead of a privilege.

After accepting all of the help that is offered from others, I must do *my* part in Prevailing. In other words, I am committed to act in order to sustain.

Here are five action-commitments which have been helpful to me:

1. Look for Christ and His Solution.
2. Use your sense of humor; decide to be of good humor.
3. Try to live in day-tight compartments.
4. Give your best efforts with the best that's left.
5. Summon determination to help you deliver.

"I hate to remind you," you protest, "but you said that you would spare me those flat, trite statements. If ever I have seen an obvious truism, you have just laid *five* on me!"

Taken as they stand, you are probably right. If I would say to you, "Do those things and all will be well," you would be justified in protesting the use of platitudes.

What I mean, however, is simply this: Those five statements represent *my* part in countering those three difficulties that *I* listed. The list is a proven recipe, a blend that has worked before in meeting *my* problems. Whether you want to use them to confront your own difficulties is your decision.

In order to be even more specific about *how* each commitment aids in the solution of specific problems such as we listed, each of the five is next spotlighted; and how it meets one or more difficulties is discussed.

1. Look for Christ and His Solution.

The decision for personal action from old Number One that obviously can affect all three of my listed problems is the action commitment named "Look for Christ and His Solution."

Then I got to thinking, "How foolish to attempt in a few sentences to describe the Solution that Jesus Christ has for my problems." No way! All I can really suggest is how stubborn a human soul and spirit can be. Look at it this way:

I think of Jesus Christ as Savior, Creator, Great Physician, and yes, even my Friend. That Solution of His that I should seek is that same Holy Spirit that I talked about earlier—the Comforter, Companion, and Spirit of Truth.

Given this combination which has power over all things, isn't it ironic that any one of those three difficulties should ever trouble me at all? Especially since I have turned all of my problems over to Him.

It's even more puzzling since I have received answers from Strength and Wisdom which are fantastically greater than mine. Somehow though, the spirit-soul parts, otherwise known as "self," take control and strongly resist trusting power that can't actually be seen.

Rather than dealing with puzzles, however, let's zero in on what often happens when specific problems are "turned over to Him." I've often been told to "cast all your cares upon Him," but seldom have I been shown how to do it.

The main part of "being" that I must use in seeking Christ and His Solution is my *will*. It is not important whether that will is part of Soul or Spirit. The vital fact is that the Inner Me acts, "willing" or committing the problems to Christ.

In my particular case today I assign Him all the weakness that goes with MS (the "body" problem), all the impatience that is bothering me (the "soul" difficulty), and the lack of trust that is troubling my spirit. And then I just wait.

"Sounds reasonable," you say. "Do you get an answer in a minute, an hour, or a day? And when do you feel the peace that He promises?"

I don't necessarily have *any* answer when I want it; nor do I always "feel" it when it comes. But I have done what He told me to do, and He promised to hear me.

My usual reason for that "blank wall" feeling is one which many Christians have in common. Even though I turn over all those problems to the Highest Power, there is still enough of self-will to think, argue, and hold on to all or part of what I just gave to the Holy Spirit.

Put another way, I still have some of those problems that I "turned over to God" by a commitment of my will because I *pulled them back* as if they were too precious to give away.

Truthfully, if I could recognize the answers from "Look for Christ and His Solution," there might be no problems at all.

2. Use Your Sense of Humor;
   Decide To Be of Good Humor

Somewhat surprisingly, listed second is the action-commitment to use (encourage) my sense of humor and to adopt an attitude of good humor. There is really more to it than "funny ha-ha" and a taped-on smile. There is definitely a problem-solving, therapeutic benefit from the combination.

Laughing in general and *laughing at myself* in particular punctures my balloon of self-satisfaction and imagined importance. Strangely enough, deflating the ego is sometimes necessary so that beneficial nourishment can replace hot air.

That truth ties closely to the second part of the commitment to be of good humor, another name for being happy. Lincoln once observed, "A fellow is about as happy as he decides that he is going to be." That simple statement certainly applies to those with chronic illness.

"Humph!" you say, "it's easy to see you don't have any of *my* problems."

Maybe not, but let's check how this action-commitment affects those three specific personal difficulties. First, the problem of impatience which is troubling Soul. What I must soothe inside me are the emotions which are constantly changing and challenging.

Impatience is simply the "now" name for all negative feelings. Brothers to impatience are discontent, jealousy, anxiety, and any other destructive emotion that clamors for attention. Now I call up a marvelous discovery—the superb "emotion tranquilizer" of laughter and good humor.

The exciting fact is that *no* negative emotion which I have can maintain its strength and overriding seriousness when I laugh at it. Impatience may not always be solved, but it is at least softened by laughter and good humor.

Next, remember that the body is influenced by the Soul. When the negative influences in the Soul are under control, the way is open for positive change in the Body part. It sometimes seems as if "I Give Up" is replaced by "Let's Get On with It!"

Finally, I've found that my spirit is more hospitable to the Holy Spirit when there is joy inside of me. I recently looked at the large number of times that the word *joy* appears in the Bible. I remember too that Christ said He came that I might have a more abundant life; that if I did things His way, my joy would be full; and that His first miracle of turning water into wine was on the joyous occasion of a wedding feast.

It doesn't seem illogical at all then that a sense of humor and the decision to be happy have always been important, and that they are basic to Prevailing in the face of what ails you and me.

3. Try to Live in Day-tight Compartments.

The third commitment to act, living in day-tight compartments, was probably first proposed around two thousand years ago. The message then offered the same inherent common sense, namely, avoid worrying about tomorrow because today's problems are quite enough, thank you.

I have found that if carried to extremes, however, "day-tight compartments" become the "head-in-the-sand" approach to difficulties. I learned in my first hospital siege that life continues "in spite of" our problems. As long as I live, I am a part of dynamic society and will interact with others.

Once oriented to these "rules of the game," though, using day-tight compartments is a plan with real merit. Reacting to difficulties such as the three I cited is shaped by three simple rules: First, yesterday is gone and can't be influenced. Second, whatever problems will come tomorrow will be met then, not today. Third, deal only with *today's* problems *today.*

You may think that those simple rules are too basic to consider. As for me, when I consciously use them they are better than a sleeping pill; and they lead to peace of soul.

This third commitment works for me in a manner similar to results from using the first two parts of the five-part blend. All three of the difficulties—with body, with soul, and with

spirit—are overcome in part by dealing with only one day's
dose of MS, impatience, and lack of trust.

4. Give Your Best Efforts with the Best That's Left.
The effects of my particular Pale Pony have shifted all the
way from a strange tingling in my hand to complete paralysis
of my legs up to apparent recovery (remission) back progressively in diminished mobility to required use of a wheelchair when I work. Whatever the actual effects though, there
has always been a great deal of "go" left.

Now this emotion may be called "drive" or "determination"
if you prefer. The name is not important; but for me, using
it has led to achievement instead of confinement, to satisfaction
rather than boredom. Even more important, I believe that every
person who is chronically ill has "go" in varying amounts.

Early I began to use this built-in drive. Maybe it was in-
herited; maybe it was learned; perhaps it was a gift. No matter
—using what I had *at each particular time,* I was able to return
to work, to go back to college, to teach, to enjoy parties and
sports activities, to write a book. It's not so much *what* I did;
the important thing is that I used what I had left at the time.

Like the first three action-commitments, this fourth one
affects each of the three troubled "people parts." Beginning with
Soul, which is favorably influenced by the calming knowledge
that I am using all of me (no matter how much there *was* of
me before), there is usually a ripple effect upon Spirit. Body
is then more capable of recovery.

5. Summon Determination to Help You Deliver.
The last commitment to act is to call up determination. Even
though other people have probably done much more with their
determination, I have personally used the emotion often enough
to know it well.

This last commitment is closely tied to the preceding one to
do your best with what's left, but it may reinforce any other
decision. Determination, an emotion that I feel stems from my
inner spirit, fills many varied needs.

For instance, after an earlier decision to look for help from
Christ, determination may take the guise of "persistence" until

I find His Solution. Then again it might become "patience" when I need it most. It might even be thought of as a catalyst, an ingredient that leads to action.

The end result of using all five of these action-commitments to face the three difficulties that I told you about was just as you might suppose. I experienced *victory* over effects of MS upon Body, of impatience upon Soul, and of lack of trust upon Spirit.

No, not a victory that forever solves my problems, but *a victory for the day I am living right now.*

That last question of yours is finally answered. And we "hold" in Prevailing.

PART THREE

Watching Him

Introduction

I am Ronald's wife, Myra Sue.

Ronald's illness is definitely not my favorite topic of conversation. As a matter of fact, I really don't even like to talk about it. But I've been asked more than a few times to express my feelings about our Pale Pony and my reactions to it.

The Pale Pony has always been very hard for me to deal with. Imagine my feelings toward an unwanted, uninvited "guest" that has been around for about fourteen years. As you would think, trying to explain my innermost thoughts and personal experiences about the Pony is quite painful. But after misgivings, prayer, encouragement, and more prayer, sharing those feelings is what this last section of the book is all about.

Please understand that I don't pretend to be an example that anyone should follow. All that I even hope to do is to share the way I feel. Simply put, perhaps putting my thoughts on paper might help someone, somewhere.

In chapter 10, "Foundations," I tell of personal and family background. As my memory leads me, we jump from courtship and marriage to children to religious training.

The rest of my part of the book is a description of changes as I saw them come with the Pale Pony. You will quickly see that those "Foundations" that I told you about were tested, shaken, but proven. Without them, I don't know what I would have done. Heaven knows, *with* them I went through enough.

I've found firsthand that the indirect effects of chronic illness —watching one step away—can be as painful as any chronic illness. Even more, I have met my own Pale Pony by being there.

Finally, I'd like to share with you certain very strong feelings. They may not solve anyone else's problems, but they help me cope with the Pale Pony.

10

Foundations

The rain chattered as it bounced off the roof of our flat-topped home in Oxford. After arrangements were completed for our regular afternoon bridge game, I settled comfortably in my favorite chair to read. Suddenly I looked up from my book and stared past the patio toward the tall green trees bathing in the steady rain.

A descriptive phrase had caused my mind to leap across six hundred miles and then backward in time by about thirty years. I no longer saw the cool, crisp Mississippi scene. Instead I relived what happened there on that hot July day in Ranger, Texas.

The images were so vivid, and the memory so sweet that I cried.

Getting Together

My mother and I had just whipped into the Texaco service station located on the corner of "downtown" Ranger, Texas. Our car was hot; we were tired because of our afternoon drive from Olney; and I was anxious to get home to shower and don my "cowgirl" outfit for the annual rodeo parade that night.

My heart skipped a beat when I noticed Ronald Pruet sitting on the Coke box in the shade. Then it flip-flopped when I saw him hop off and start toward me, smiling all the way. He was very friendly and quite curious. When I told him that

I would be riding in the parade, he laughed and said that he and Prince, his white horse, would see me later then.

My excitement was quite normal because, you see, Ronald had been my steady during our senior year at Ranger High School. "Steady" in this case meant that he and I had at least one date each weekend, that I cheered mostly for him at football games (he was a tackle, and I was head cheerleader), and that I was his regular date at school dances and other "special" occasions. But then he went off to college at Texas Tech in Lubbock, while I enrolled at the local junior college. That separation led to such a devastating quarrel that we had not spoken to each other for two years.

Yet mysteriously, even then I knew deep inside me that he was mine and that someday—*someday*—I would marry him.

When Mother and I drove away from the station, I turned to her and said cheerfully, "Ronald is going to call me and ask for a date! He didn't tell me that—I just know."

"And if he does," she asked, knowing that my current flame and I had been talking seriously about marriage, "what are you going to do?"

"I'm going to go with him."

He did call, and I went—again and again. More often than before, Ronald and I were together, doing all the summer things that most kids in small towns do to be near each other. We swam, rode horses and then bicycles, went on picnics, played tennis. And fell in love again.

A short tale about two young people and how they were attracted to each other? Yes, but all of those words, no matter how I put them together, fall far short in describing my feelings about Ronald. Let me tell you a little more.

Even before we started dating again, I imagined how I would act if I saw Ronald at the next dance, what I would say when we "happened" to meet, or even Ronald's reaction to the special dress I would wear. Call it what you care to, but I *knew* who I wanted. As a matter of fact, I had even prayed about it. He was the only one that I could imagine in my picture of Happiness.

Oh, I can reluctantly admit now that I *might* have been oversold on him then, that he *might* not have been perfect, and that life *might* have a few questions that he couldn't answer. I sure didn't feel that way then though. And you know what? After twenty-six years of being married to Ronald, I feel the same way today, only much more so.

Beginning, I suppose, when that gawky young man jumped off that Coke box in Ranger, we started a structure of love and respect that didn't peak early and then shrink. Instead, those mutual feelings have grown each year. On a cold winter's night in Lubbock, less than two years after we started dating that summer, he proposed marriage to me. The following summer he started work for an oil company, and we were married in August.

Like every newly married couple, possible problems were never considered. "How could there be anything but happiness in Camelot?"

Suddenly the answer to that question came to me as if it were spotlighted: "Very naturally and quite unexpectedly, that's how!"

Then I thought, "Ronald and I have climbed a lot rougher road than we expected when we started together, and the top of the mountain does not even seem close."

Three Foundations

Pausing now to look back at where we've been, I can see that we've passed through several dark valleys. What's more, I notice three main strengths in my marriage that have helped me get this far on our journey. My first foundation came from love that we added to living together, the next from deeper roots with children, and the last from religious training as a child.

It's not so much that I have attained the peak in my struggles with the Pony. It is rather that I wouldn't be as high on the hill as I am now without those three foundations.

How do you prepare for cares in Camelot?

Add Love to Living Together

In sickness and in health,
From this day forward
Until death us do part.

I don't suppose that anyone starts a marriage by planning how to handle problems she can't foresee. Those day-to-day problems were quite enough for me, thank you. We turned peace into panic at home pretty often when we "adjusted" (I'll be honest—"argued" is a better word). We certainly didn't plan on any bigger struggles.

As I look back now, I see that we bristled regularly about problems that we ourselves created in living together. You know —those important things like "not going out" or maybe about seeing my family when *I* wanted to. "Big" problems.

What I didn't realize or even remotely imagine then was the fact that our adjusting to each new problem was actually building a strong marriage, one capable of coping with unimagined problems. Problems for both of us that *we* didn't originate.

Now I am not going to launch into a "how to" about making a good marriage, but I will share some thoughts that the apostle Paul offered a long time ago in the Love Chapter in Corinthians. He said, "Three things will last: faith, hope, and love, but the greatest of these is love."

Don't get me wrong. Ronald and I have been far from perfect in applying this truth in our marriage. But I have been thinking—we have always had faith in each other; we have supported each other with hope. Most of all, the love that we started with has grown and matured. And that's important!

What this means to me now, after we've met the Pale Pony, is simply this: Preparing for unforeseen problems is very difficult. Part of our preparation probably came from lessons learned in reacting to smaller conflicts.

One of the most important things for then—and now—is adding love to living together.

Deeper Roots—Three Children

Married life without children was fun. Three years without

babies passed quickly, and we wouldn't trade for experiences we had then. But we had always planned to have children "after a while."

We agreed that three years was long enough for "after a while." Happy result—our first child was born. As a matter of fact, we were so pleased that we had visions of four of the same! We did drop that desired number to three though. After the third son was born, Ronald and I agreed, "Three really *is* a crowd!" Like any busy mother with a family that size, I could tell you in great detail, complete with many pictures, about the virtues and brainpower of child number one, Ronnie; leave a gap or two in describing Rick the live-wire number two; and then search for *that* picture of Brent, son three.

I stand in awe, however, whenever I pause, look at all three, and realize that those men—and that's what they are now, three men—are part of my family. And that they actually wouldn't be here on earth unless Ronald and I loved each other.

Several facts about them are clear to me now. First, those sons cannot doubt that each is a *family* member and is loved (though often embattled) by his parents and brothers. Second, all three have been affected in varying degrees by the Pale Pony. Third, each one is very definitely an individual, influenced by mother and dad but encouraged to think for himself and to assume responsibility.

I confess that I do not know all of the innermost thoughts of Ron, Rick, and Brent; nor can I learn all that they feel about our Pale Pony. I really can only imagine.

I can easily recall all of the fun times we had together before; but then again, we have a closeness now that is heart warming. They seem to accept gracefully those changes that were dictated by MS.

As I think back about problems that we have faced in the past fourteen years, I can truthfully say that our sons have added purpose, stability, and love to our family. Yes, they have added deep roots and strength to the Ronald Pruets of Oxford.

Train Up a Child

My third foundation, religious training as a child, might seem sort of pretentious. You understand—as if claiming I've done so well with my problems because I have always been a good Christian. I am quick to say that such a meaning is not at all what I imply.

Foundations support what you and I build on them. What's more, they are laid down even before we start building. We don't "renew" foundations for they are already there, supporting whatever kind of life we shape.

Religious training as a child was an important part of my growing up. Call it part of my heritage. What I do with that training—use it, build on it, pass it on, lean on it, or forget it—is my responsibility, and it seems to me, my challenge.

The most powerful and loving Christians that I have ever known were my grandmother and grandfather Gray. As a child, I used to spend at least two weeks every summer with them in Olney, the north central Texas town where they lived. The routine that I joined so willingly doesn't sound exciting or even entertaining, but what it did for me one summer needs to be told. That too is part of my heritage.

As always, every Sunday morning we all went to Sunday school and then to service in the big Methodist church. After dinner I went with them Sunday afternoon to one and sometimes two missionary Methodist churches in nearby hamlets. That night we returned to the church services in Olney, just as we would the following Wednesday night for prayer meeting.

It sounds like it would get very stale very fast. It would have except for one big thing: mama and papa were *happy*—so happy that it was contagious! Only by being with them then would you fully understand what I mean.

The routine was regular, except when week-long revivals were scheduled. Then we went to church every night. Special things happened to me that summer in such a revival, when I was eleven years old.

I remember the experience much more than the messages. I had gone every night to hear the fervent evangelistic preacher, listened to his altar calls when he pled for decisions for Christ, and said regularly to myself, "Maybe tomorrow...." Then I would go home with mama and papa.

Finally the week was nearly over. Strangely, I remember that I wore my aunt's red tennis shoes that night to the climax service. As we all stood to sing the last hymn, the preacher called for the unsaved to "step out for Jesus," and I knew he was talking to me. I edged one borrowed shoe out into the aisle, hesitated, and then pulled it back. The wavering continued for at least three verses of the invitation hymn; then I summoned courage, pushed out into the aisle, and rushed forward to the front.

At the end of the service mama came running down the aisle with papa right behind her. Tears were streaming down her face. I was surprised to see mama cry and hear her say, "I'm so glad you decided! We've been praying for you."

I didn't know they had been doing that. Yes, I had seen them pray, but I had no idea that it was for me.

But the greatest thrill came that night when I was alone. Jesus was so real to me that I saw Him in the Garden. Just like the song, He talked with me and showed me the dew on the roses. He told me that I was His and that He loved me very much.

There have been only a few times that He has been as close to me as He was then. But this much is true: No matter how I "feel" about the fact, the foundation was laid, and it's just as real today as it was then.

Inspirations

The strength that I can gain in coping with "now" problems from the Pale Pony is much like the water in a deep cistern that mama and papa had in their backyard in Olney. At the beginning of my annual summer visit I would often forget that the cistern was there.

Yet when I needed a cool drink of water and asked her for it, mama would remind me of the cistern. My part was to lower the bucket, fill it, and draw it up. The water's part was just being there.

So it is, I believe, with strength from Christianity.

Oh, that sounds so easy. But let me tell you something. It is *not* so simple and trite as it sounds.

I believe with all my heart in the reality of Jesus and that He loves me. Yet I still have to watch the effects of the Pale Pony on Ronald. Surely I've convinced you by now that what happens to him hurts me too. Sometimes I am certain that my pain, though one step away, is greater than his.

Yes, I've learned all too well that God's children are not exempt from troubles. Believe me, I've prayed that they would go away. Then I remember how Jesus ended the Sermon on the Mount. He told of storms that would come against houses which are built either foolishly on sand or wisely on bed-rock foundations. Just because its foundation is solid rock, that house is *not* spared from storms.

Finally I thought again of the strength I draw from my three main foundations: love in living together, deeper roots with children, and early religious training. Enough to prevail.

But there's even more. I have a sacred promise of help from One who said He loves me. He has Conquered whatever direct and indirect problems the Pale Pony brings us. *More* than prevailing.

11

Struggles

I tried to fill in some of the blank spaces about me and the way I think with that written conversation that we just had. You remember—that glimpse of Ronald's and my courtship, our marriage, and all that talk about the three foundations which are most important to me.

I didn't share it to suggest that I am an example to follow or that you should have similar experiences. Rather than either of these purposes, it serves as background to separate but connected reactions to the Pale Pony that I tell you about. Perhaps you will better understand the reasons for my responses. I know that I still search for answers.

Too, I make this point very emphatically. What I have been through is very definitely not a "personal trials formula" which others could (or would even want to) copy, expecting solutions to the indirect problems from the Pony. Besides, I certainly wouldn't wish these experiences on anyone!

Nevertheless, I tell about them because I firmly believe that others who share the Stand-Beside-and-Watch living pattern will mysteriously be strengthened when they read of another's battles.

And, really now, that's the main purpose of this section, isn't it?

Myra Meets His Pony

We were three years into what had been promised as the "Soaring Sixties" in sandy west Texas. Then Ronald told me that the oil business had gone sour; that the coin-op we had helped finance in Odessa had gone broke; and that the new leasing company he was organizing in Midland was not off the ground yet.

I remember thinking, "If what we're doing is 'soaring,' I think I'll settle for an atomic bomb shelter."

Besides those business woes however, something else had been wrong, off and on, for about two years at home in Midland. Something that I couldn't put my finger on. I didn't know then that the Pale Pony had moved in with us.

More and more often, Ronald was not himself. He was nervous, impatient, and changeable in mood without warning. I knew that he was under a strain from business problems, but he had never before reacted this way when he was faced with difficulties.

For example, he would come home from the office, everything apparently normal and happy. He would laugh and wrestle with the boys. Then suddenly, as if a curtain fell over him, he would push the happy boys away, showing irritation to both them and me.

When that happened, something like a bewildering, invisible wall would form between him and me. I couldn't even talk to him as before. On my side of the "wall" I found myself trying to protect Ronald from the turmoil—all the things that happen in any home with three lively young boys. But no matter what I did or didn't do, there was a strange new tension between us.

I decided that he was on the verge of a nervous breakdown. Understand that he looked outwardly—to others at least— just like he always did. His "symptoms" as I described them were not always there. What's more, the warning sign that seemed to be more important to him at the time was often less important to me. As a result, both of us were puzzled about what the problem actually was.

To find an answer Ronald had more than one physical examination. First our family doctor in Midland, then one in Odessa, finally another in Abilene. All the time, of course, without any outward sign to anyone else but me that something was wrong.

Putting it briefly—we couldn't name the Pony. I wasn't even sure then that I could live with the label when we found out what it was.

In my uncertainty I drifted back toward a somewhat neglected foundation. Oh, the Lord was not exactly a stranger to me, but He was not my bosom buddy either. I knew the Bible well from earlier exposure though, had various responsibilities in Sunday school, and I did pray occasionally. I came to realize that I needed help—more than I could get from once-in-a-while calls for send-this-too needs.

I set aside a time for regular Bible study and prayer. I'm an early morning person; so I set the alarm for 5:30 A.M. At first it was a struggle, but later it became a habit to arise early and then go into the den for sunrise prayer and Bible study. Before long I began to be comfortable with Jesus as a personal friend. We shared ideas every morning.

Starting gently, He introduced me to a different set of truths and values. In comparison, the ones that I had seemed very frail and shabby. Too, He caused me to look at my problems from a different point of view.

I began to realize that little else was really important in this world if my dearest loved ones didn't have health. What's more, I found from our morning exchanges that nothing else was important if I didn't have the Lord as my best friend.

Solid truths? Yes, I learned these lessons very well—intellectually. But I had a hard time working these facts into the way I lived *all day long*.

One spring night that year, long after the whole family had gone to sleep, I lay there, wide-eyed and mind-racing. That whole day, particularly after Ronald got home, had been very painful and trying. I got out of bed, closed the door, and went into the living room. For the first time since I was a little girl,

I got down on my knees and began to pray with all my heart and soul.

In deep agony I cried and talked with Jesus. I told Him that none of unrealized goals in life mattered any more—big houses, flashy cars, fur coats, swimming pools. Nothing mattered but our family and Ronald's health! In the same breath I surrendered *my* plans and manipulations to Him.

Yes, I gave my will to God. He accepted it, and I fell back exhausted.

Two weeks later Ronald checked into the hospital in Abilene. Doctors there diagnosed his mysterious illness as multiple sclerosis. The shadow that had hung over our lives for nearly two years materialized. I met our Pale Pony.

The Lord had prepared me for it. Earlier in our married life I had been a very dependent person. Because of this trait I was surprised when I found an inner strength that had not been there before.

During those weeks that Ronald was in the Abilene hospital, what Jesus told His disciples in the last few days of His public ministry became very real to me. It meant so much to think about the promise in these words: "Have faith and doubt not— you can say to this mountain, 'Move over into the ocean!' and it will. You can get anything that you ask in prayer, if you believe."

The mountain is still there as I write, but a lot of the boulders were moved aside.

Moving on to a more painful experience, Ronald and I decided to go to the Mayo Clinic in Rochester, Minnesota. Though we really couldn't see how we'd get to the clinic, we nursed a faint hope for better news from the supposedly most expert doctors in the country.

With remarkable speed our decision to go led us to the "latest word" there about multiple sclerosis in 1963. Much to my dismay, however, when the doctors made their diagnosis they added many pessimistic predictions.

They said to Ronald, "You will be lucky if you make it to a wheelchair. Your life expectancy is not very long." And many other distressing things. What they told him caused Ronald to break for the first and only time! He was so upset at the thought of being a helpless burden to the boys and me.

Then a few words that Paul said to church members in Corinth became full of meaning to me. Without them I don't think I could have made it. He said to them—and to me, "I want your faith to stand in the power of God, not in the wisdom of men."

At that time and in that place, I was given strength and peace when there was no encouragement from anywhere else— not from doctors, not from Ronald, not from family, not from circumstances. Looking back, I *know* that He looks after His children, no matter what the problem.

The next day after we heard the diagnosis, I packed our bags and we went back to "our hospital" in Abilene, Texas. Within a month Ronald was able to walk again. He checked out of the hospital and went back to full-time work in Midland. The summer was over, and our life had changed.

Myra Meets Her Own Pony

I've made that earlier experience sound so easy—as if we really didn't have a thing to worry about. Nothing could be further from the truth! In addition to everyday problems that come with tending to a family (and paying for it), I carried in the back of my mind a haunting picture of a helpless Ronald in a hospital. It was a heavy load.

Added to that weight was what family, friends, doctors— it seemed like *everyone*—told me. They said that I must learn how to earn a living and go to work, because in my situation. . . ???? I had never done those things in the fourteen years we had been married, but I began to cast around as soon as we got home because "they" said I must.

Lo and behold, I found that the easiest and best work for a woman with young children was teaching school. What's more, I learned that the psychology courses I took fifteen years earlier counted toward a Texas teacher's certificate. The Lord had looked after me, it seemed, even when I didn't have enough sense to ask Him.

I was very fortunate to land a job that very fall, even though I had never before dreamed of teaching the fourth grade. However, the strain of studying for my new job, being a mother, taking refresher courses, and watching my husband's recovery like a hawk was almost too much to bear.

After nearly two years with those loads, I was so relieved when Ronald decided that he would go back to school for more training. He wanted to find a better way to provide for the boys and me—even if some day it might be from a wheelchair. We prayed to God for open doors if this move was His will. As an answer, we found ourselves in Austin almost before we knew we were there, where Ronald enrolled as a graduate student in Texas University.

My full-time job in Austin was to keep the boys in line and to maintain peace and quiet, as far as possible, for my student husband. Life at first there was much better, and my inner pressures were eased considerably (I thought).

The Pony, however, stayed with us.

Ronald pushed himself unmercifully; so much that I was increasingly worried about his getting enough rest. My concern was multiplied when I remembered the bad things that doctors had said about fatigue and MS.

I hadn't planned to do it, but I found myself "doctoring" Ronald! If *I* thought he was not walking as well as he should, or if *I* imagined that he was "worn out," *I* would secretly call his Abilene doctor for advice. Then *I* would tell Ronald that the dosage in the shots that he was taking had to be changed. Of course *I* was the one who gave him the shots.

I found that I spent more and more time watching, watching, watching. And I was tired.

I was so weary then—nearly five years since Ronald was in the hospital—that I sometimes let my imagination take charge. When that happened, I wished I could be alone in a boat, lying down, floating in a sea of blackness—where there was nothing ... nothing that could disturb me. Things were closing in on me, and I had no place to run!

One Monday at lunch with a friend, we had a glass—maybe

two—of dry wine. I felt light-headed, calmer, and very relaxed. After we finished, I came home, crawled into bed to rest, and then strangely could not muster the strength to prepare dinner for my hungry brood. Hamburgers that night for everyone— but me! I slept.

As a matter of fact I slept for three days and nights until Thursday, when I roused to ask Ronald to cancel a regular appointment at the beauty parlor. That move, plus the sleep, was so unusual that he finally realized that something was really wrong. How he knew what to do, I still don't understand. Instead of phoning a regular doctor, Ronald called a psychiatrist and made an appointment for the next day.

I didn't know what to expect at my appointment the next morning, but I didn't protest going. I remember the dress I wore, though what we said in that first meeting escapes me. Whatever, Dr. Muncie told Ronald that I needed to check into Holy Cross, a psychiatric hospital. Ronald didn't much want me to go, but he knew I needed help. That same day he made the arrangements, and I moved into my room.

Relief! Relief! Relief! Lively as a child celebrating Christmas, I came to life there! With great gusto I did all the therapy things that they had for the patients—square dancing, decoupage, guitar lessons—and celebrating my fortieth birthday with my new friends like I was six years old.

I liked it there without any stress and strain; without any problems with Ronald or worry about his studying for examinations; without concerns over the boys or *anything!* I had found my boat, sailed blissfully onto the black sea, and arrived on the shores of Wonder Land—no Pale Pony even thought of. Ronald and the boys were bewildered. To them I didn't look sick or act sick, and they wanted me to come home. I didn't want to go!

Dr. Muncie finally convinced Ronald that I was very ill, and that in order to be well I had to come to terms with myself. Doing that meant I had to face who I was, what I was made of, and what life was all about.

After a week in Wonder Land, the doctor put me to sleep

with the "truth serum." This treatment was a mirror that let me look clearly at the weak, dependent, sickened soul that was there.

It made me angry! What's more, I was angry with God! I remember spending an entire afternoon crying and shaking my fist at God, asking why?

> Oh, why have You done this to me? I am a Christian! I am a Sunday school teacher! Ronald is good, kind, gentle! Why is he ill? My family needs me, and I can't help them!!

I was hysterical and could not stop crying until they gave me a shot to calm me. When I awakened, I realized where I was. It wasn't in Wonder Land—I was in a living hell!

I felt as if my life had been a fragile vase, that God had hurled me against a brick wall, and that I had shattered into a million pieces. I was left lying there with no one caring.

Gradually though, beginning the next day, "someone" started picking up the pieces to make me a whole person again. It was a strange and frightening experience.

My doctor came each morning. We talked, and it seemed then as if he stepped on the broken pieces of my vase. Almost every afternoon Dr. Ralph Smith, the wonderful minister from my church, would come to visit. He knew about problems with broken vases. Slowly, very slowly the pieces were picked up. Though they didn't fit too well, they were at least laid out and ready to go together.

After many morning visits, Dr. Muncie finally suggested what had happened to me. He said that life as I saw it came complete with a Prince Charming, and his name was Ronald. Ronald rode a white horse and carried a shining sword to defend and protect me. But one day Prince Charming got sick and fell off his horse. I had never recovered from his fall.

Maybe the doctor was right—I'm still not sure. But this much I found out—I had run so hard from Ronald's Pale Pony that I had been trapped by my own. And it was vicious.

When Dr. Muncie kicked me out of what began as Wonder

Land, I started the long, slow journey back to mental health. And believe me, there's a steep mountain to climb to get there from where I was.

Let me tell those of you who have never been mentally ill, "recovering" is no picnic. Those of you who have been there will recognize the problems. When I left the hospital, I was not well. It was as if I had been through a special kind of surgery. My "surgeon," Dr. Muncie, had sliced me open—top to bottom—and then quickly stitched the gaping wounds closed. Next he patted me on the arm and told me to walk unassisted back to where I lived.

In the weeks that followed my one-month stay in Wonder Land-Living Hell I returned periodically to my psychiatrist. My feelings toward him ranged from respect and gratitude to pure hatred. Yet somehow I started to improve.

I was going through a long, agonizing process which Ronald and my boys didn't understand. You see, most of the time I looked so normal, so like before, that they couldn't see the mental stitches; nor could they understand the reasons for many of my actions. They couldn't imagine why sometimes I would stay in bed, pull the covers over my head, and refuse to get up.

I would lie there and pray to die! During times like that I would have gladly traded Ponies with Ronald.

Soon Dr. Muncie told me that I should take a couple of summer courses at the University—any course would do. "Therapy," you know. I did as he said, enjoying not one minute of it. After he saw some improvement (maybe he imagined it), he then prescribed a job—regular work at regular times.

Ronald was writing his dissertation; so I was faced with one more full year in Austin. I *was* better, and I *am* a good teacher. Solution: get a teaching job.

It was ironic that in a city of 300,000 people the only job that I could find and qualify for was as a third grade teacher in the Texas State School for the Deaf. The children were beautiful, smart, and could read lips well—but each was handicapped by his own Pale Pony. And they were taught by a teacher who was often plagued by her own.

Teaching them did help all of us, but there were times that my drive across Austin from my house to that job seemed to be pure torture. The year started slowly, and there were, I confess, too many times that I was just not able to push myself across the city to work.

Two things happened, however, that speeded my climb out of the miry pit.

After I had been teaching for about two months, the Shrine Circus came to town. All of the patients in state institutions were invited to attend. I was walking my deaf students into the circus just as the bus from the State Mental Hospital arrived. The mental patients filed slowly, almost haltingly from the bus. One man in their group must have thought that he was to go in with me.

When I guided him back to the other mental patients, I looked at his expression and at the faces of his companions. I saw vacant, hopeless stares from bodies that seemed tragically like empty shells. It was much worse than anything I had seen at Holy Cross.

My stomach tightened and a chill ran down my spine. Right then and there I made up my mind to work harder at getting well. I made a vow to myself that I would *not* cry each morning at the breakfast table; I would no longer beg Ronald to let me stay home. I *would* go to school willingly and fight the urge to go back to bed.

Yes, this incident speeded my recovery—I was scared!

The second happening that lifted me was when Ronald told me about our job offer at the University of Mississippi. It had the elements that we wanted for each member of our family.

I fell in love with the town, the University, and the new opportunities. I saw Dr. Muncie for the last time.

Surely the stitches were healed, and my Pony was left behind in Austin when we moved to Oxford after school was over.

Yet—was it really?

12

From Crashing to Coping

Back in the mainstream again! And I didn't even test it with one toe to check the temperature. We five transplanted Texans jumped right into our new places in the Old South.

Oxford was great—all that we had hoped for. The boys were ready to be somewhere they could really call "home" after their daddy finished four years in graduate school. Ron began his senior year in high school, Rick the eighth grade, and Brent the fifth. Their first year in school here, 1969-1970, was when integration was enforced in Mississippi. A lot of reaction but actually no trouble in the end. By mid-term the boys were adjusted.

We moved into an old (but not ante-bellum) white house on the tree-lined street going north from the downtown square. The peace that was a fixture in that home was better than any doctor's prescription. Although the boys couldn't understand their mother's troubles, they loved me; and we were all ready for the soothing calm we found in Oxford.

At the risk of sounding like an advertisement for small-town southern living, I want to touch on how well our move here met family needs for acceptance and activity. For instance, Ronald found out that he loved teaching, although he had never done it before. At the same time, the boys met new friends, just as I did—and they welcomed us. Maybe it's because we openly liked them—maybe because we were new and not too strange. Whatever it was, somehow we felt like we had "moved back home."

Oxford is a football-, bridge-, and party-town. It didn't take me any time at all to shift gears from "student's wife" to "professor's wife." All of us were more comfortable in our new roles. We really enjoyed watching the Ole Miss football team win with Archie Manning. We joined the caravans to Jackson for "home games" 160 miles south of Oxford and then were delighted with the custom of "Open house" here after local contests. Yes, life was a lot more relaxing—full of fun and good times.

We chose a church that seemed to offer the most for all of us, and the whole family joined. Even though I usually took part in the worship services, I confess that I did not even look for the closeness to God that had been mine before. Dr. Muncie had told me that I was full of hostility. Most couldn't see it, but it was there in force. Without planning it, I drifted further from God, and more of my anger toward Him began to surface. Less church, no Bible, more rebellion.

Though I didn't seek God, He was looking out for me in spite of my rebellious ways. He gave me some precious friends in Oxford that could see how much I needed Him. What's more, they prayed long and hard for me. I am amazed by the fact too that there was so much love directed my way by "friends of my friends"—people that had never laid eyes on Myra Sue Pruet.

And you know what? Heartfelt prayer does change things! Before very long I joined certain of those friends in weekly prayer meetings. When my fellowship was reopened, I caught a glimpse of the peace that He promised.

"Surely," I thought, "I must be doing what He intends now. I think I can see His will for me and mine."

In the meantime, however, all was not well. I watched Ronald closely and could see that he was getting weaker instead of stronger. When we first came to Oxford, he could and would walk a mile every night—up and down some pretty steep hills.

Slowly but certainly, his condition deteriorated. Soon he walked only every other night because the mile took so much out of him—then every third night—then not at all.

Ronald's next physical exercise was to swim in a heated pool that we had access to at Ole Miss. This early morning dip seemed to be helpful, and he was faithful in keeping it up. After a while, he told me that the walk from the pool to the car when he had finished his swim exhausted him. He tried to do more until one doctor finally told him to use the energy that he had for what must be done—walking from the car to his office, his office to classes, and inside our house.

As you might imagine, by now I was wringing my hands. That old inner fear began gnawing at me again—I needed help! I found it by taking part in a second prayer group, the one that prayed for me before they had even seen me. I found God's outstretched arms and realized that though we are without faith and trust, the Lord still waits for His erring children. For a while I lived in the comfort that a strayed calf must have felt when it was found.

But still the problem did not go away. We all prayed for a miracle—but no miracle came.

I asked myself why, and then searched for things that might stand in the way. More prayer needed? more Bible study? more dedication? more submission? for me? for Ronald? more confession? more praise? help from more dedicated Christians? prayer in tongues? I tried first one and then another and then combinations of them all. Still no results that I could see.

Then for the first time since the Pale Pony had been identified, I took a deeper, honest look at my own personal life, and this is what I saw: Ronald Pruet was the best thing that had ever happened to me. I loved him deeply—with all my being. Yet because of what was happening, I was truly aggrieved, brokenhearted, and in deep anguish. In my pain, time telescoped for me; for I could see Ronald's life slipping away. And I resented it!

When the husband, father, and breadwinner is ill, there is so much to consider. I thought, "He brings home the paycheck every month. If something happens and he can't, what am I going to do?"

Aside from loving him very much, chronic illness forces the one who stands beside to face cold, hard facts—and I was no exception. In my case there were three boys to raise, educate, and feed. On top of that was the possibility of lots of medical expense and care for the breadwinner himself. The load was too much for me to carry alone. I prayed—but I also worried.

I didn't just sit down and do nothing either! I decided to return to graduate school at Ole Miss to get a Master's degree in Guidance and Counseling. It took me a full year as a full-time student—added to what I had already done in graduate studies—to earn this degree. All the time I was doing this, I looked forward to a good paying job which would help the professor's salary make ends meet. In the back of my mind I knew that it would prepare me to take care of all of us if the need arose.

It seems sometimes that the whole world is talking about "Women's Lib." In the graduate classroom—especially in Guidance and Counseling—they discuss the job world and that women must have equal rights with men. Well, basically I'm not a "Women's Libber" because I agree with my prayer group, which was teaching submission to the husband as head of the family and what the Lord expects of a woman. The Biblical teaching and the classroom teaching were in direct conflict. I was in a quandary.

My true feelings lay with the Word of God, but I couldn't make my life to fit neatly into either category. I want to be protected and cared for. I don't have to be equal with a man. On the other hand, if I were in the "World of Work"—doing the same amount of work as a man—I would want to make as much money as he does. There you see—two conflicting views that were tearing me to pieces. Coupled with that tearing was the fact that Ronald was not getting stronger nor had his condition stabilized.

Even so, Ronald wanted me to go back to school, and the

Lord did, too. But the Lord had a different twist in His plan for our lives.

Degree in hand, I went looking for a job; but in Oxford there was nothing to be had. I was back where I started—with the exception of having bagged the Master's.

What a predicament I was in! It was like living in a maze with no right answer. One minute I could see just what the Lord was telling me to do—I was confident, full of faith and trust. The next moment I was thrust back by circumstances—watching Ronald, listening to professors, adding up the bills—into the "real" world. Being submissive, free from worry about "no job," and brave about problems with the Pale Pony—all of that was nothing but foolish folly.

I am a "doing" person, but unfortunately the more I did then, the more frantic I became. My world looked hopeless to me. I was being backed into a corner, and my Pale Pony—mental illness—had reared high on its hind legs, ready to trample me.

I escaped my turmoil every afternoon by having a good stiff drink. My five o'clock "appointment"—as I saw it then—sort of smoothed out the problems for a while. One Sunday afternoon, things looked very bleak to me. To solve it I invited some friends over for drinks and conversation. I just had to get away from my situation for a few minutes.

I didn't realize beforehand what was coming. All that I really planned was to relax, laugh, and enjoy. But the pressures that had been building up inside clamored for recognition.

After everyone left, Ronald and I were alone. Then I realized that nothing—nothing at all—had been helped. The dam broke. I began to cry, then wail, then scream! I *had* to be set free!! I could not tolerate my life style anymore; nor could I watch Ronald's life slipping away from me!!!

My Pale Pony joined Ronald's Pale Pony! Together their hooves came crashing down upon me!!

The next thing I can remember was being put in a car, hearing the voices of my family, and then everything went black.

After a while they shifted me out of the car into a wheelchair and took me somewhere I had never been before. I vaguely recall hearing Ronald comment to the boys when they put me on an elevator that it took a key to stop the elevator on my floor.

I was going to be locked up somewhere. I couldn't have cared less; so I dropped off to sleep.

After about two days of solid sleeping I was jarred awake by a dream—a vision—something so real that I get shivers even today when I tell about it. I saw myself in a courtroom alive with action and argument—and *I* was the one on trial!

Satan was the Accuser. I can't tell you what he looked like— maybe because I was afraid to watch him—but I remember what he said. He literally screamed at the Judge, "At last she belongs to me!"

Then he listed the ways that I had disappointed God, ending with a trumpet sound, "And she even tried suicide! It's plain that Myra Sue Pruet is a 'has-been' Christian that Jesus no longer wants!"

Then another voice, calmer—even stronger—took the floor. It came from Jesus, my Advocate.

He spoke to Satan, "Myra Sue does not belong to you. She is one of God's own children—one that I love very much. Lucifer, you are the father of lies! Flee from our presence! By the blood which I shed on the cross, she is protected and shall be healed."

And then the trial ended.

I can't adequately describe what it means to be defended by the Lord Himself. Nor can I explain why a few days later I still had mixed feelings about my problems. Jesus had shown me that He cares—but why didn't He take away all the things that bothered me so much?

I wouldn't blame you for being puzzled because I don't know the answer either. After all, Jesus Himself dismissed Satan— but the problems that Satan had brought stayed behind. I had believed with all my heart that God would heal Ronald. But Ronald was not better. And now to compound it all, I was in a bad way mentally.

Why Ronald?

Why me?

Days later, I found a proverb that seemed to describe the problem we faced—but it didn't tell the cure: "The spirit of a man will sustain his infirmity; but a wounded spirit, who can bear?"

I wanted to go home immediately, but Dr. Crupie and my four men knew I needed rest and treatment. Ronald called my mother to stay with them in Oxford, and they left me in the Memphis hospital. At first I was so lonely, and my heart kept reaching out for my family—very different from five years earlier in Austin. But I knew even more that I had to get myself organized and thinking straight.

None of it was easy in the month that I stayed in Memphis. The Lord made sure that I was in the proper care though, because I had a fine Christian psychiatrist. Evidence again that He cares for His children when we are in bad trouble.

As time passed I was convicted of how wrong I had been that night, and how selfish I was. I had not considered anyone but myself and had overlooked the fact that with Christ I would never be alone. Again I was broken. I understood what David meant when he prayed, "Create in me a clean heart, O God; and renew a right spirit within me. Cast me not away from thy presence, and take not thy Holy Spirit from me."

Furthermore, I began to see clearly how brokenhearted I was about Ronald's illness—how desolate and alone I felt. Then I realized that I truly am a child of God, that I must trust Him for everything, and that my faith must be strengthened. He showed me personally about the psalmist's message, "The sacrifices of God are a broken spirit. A broken and contrite heart, O God, thou wilt not despise." I gave God my broken heart and surrendered totally.

Thoughts That I Carry
And
Thoughts That Carry Me

When I came home from my hospital stay in Memphis, there was none of the withdrawing, the "hide under the covers" approach to problems, that I had gone through five years before in Texas. Instead I stepped right back into life. I cherish the support that my dear friends gave me. Their love—and their prayers—helped make a smooth return possible.

But, of course too, I had some help from my doctor. As I write this some two years after returning to Oxford, I am still on medication and see Dr. Crupie about every three months. It's not easy, but I am coping—sometimes triumphantly, sometimes from a valley.

There has been one big change though. My anger about Ronald's Pale Pony is no longer directed at God. I have learned instead to focus on the source of the Pony problems—Satan himself. I don't claim to understand why evil must "have its day," but being angry with my dearest Friend doesn't solve the riddles. I believe in divine healing; and when the Lord is ready, Ronald will be healed. More than that even, I know that I myself am totally dependent on the Lord. I believe that He cares about our problems.

Another thing I have discovered—salvation is for the here and now—not just in the by-and-by. I know too that I am a rich relative of God. I can have the abundant life that Jesus promised and have it *now*. That's one promise that I claim for each day-tight compartment I live in.

Sounds peaceful and calm, doesn't it? But sometimes negative thoughts leak into my not-so-tightly sealed compartments. For instance, one day I saw how much fun a good friend and her husband were having on trips together. Without warning a mixture of pure envy and warmed-over self-pity flooded in.

I thought, "Why couldn't Ronald and I jump into the car and run to Memphis for the day? Just doing what we would like to do—having dinner and then driving home late? Or better yet—why not a trip to Las Vegas, Hawaii, or anywhere our little hearts desired? Other people do—why not us?"

But we can't. Not enough money. Not enough strength. Not enough time. Thinking like this is a vicious, distressing circle. Thankfully, the circle is not a regular part of my life now.

Those are some of the thoughts that I carry.

Then I stepped back and looked at thoughts that carry me through some tough times—those days when I watch Ronald with his back to the wall—fighting to walk, to work, just to *be*. Many times I am frightened about what might happen. . . .

But then I come back to the fact that I love Ronald, only Ronald, with all my heart. And he loves me the same way. Others must see it, too. The other night our oldest son shared something beautiful with us. We were laughing back and forth about some of the ups and downs he had seen in his mother and dad. We said to him, "Having lived through it all with us, you will probably think several times before you ask a girl to share your life."

He turned and said quite seriously, "I'm very proud of you two, and I hope that my marriage can be as good as yours is."

I cry as I write those words because I know that in spite of everything I am very fortunate—a much-loved woman. I really do not want to walk in anyone else's shoes. I want only to be able to kick the Pale Pony of MS in the derriere. Once we are rid of him, my Pale Pony of mental illness automatically is done away with.

Then I looked again at the support that I have had from our sons. As far as the boys are concerned, I have thoughts that make me stronger. The Lord has blessed us with boys that love us; and *most* of the time (notice I didn't say *all*) they respect our opinions. Ronald has kept a steady line of communication open to them, and they use it. We've had anxious moments with each son—and will probably have more—but we have been able to discuss each separately and then go forward from there.

My very loving men have sometimes assumed the role of taking care of their parents. I appreciate it when it is offered, and a deeper love has come from their help. I'll never forget the time in Memphis when they came to me, expressed their love and affection, and assured me that life without me would be grim. You know what? Out of tragic circumstances has come a deeper, more sustaining family relationship.

Finally, regardless of the problems that the Ponies bring, I am more peaceful and relaxed now. This improvement is because I know the Holy Spirit is at work in my daily affairs. We exchange ideas early every day. I depend on morning worship for guidance for the rest of the day and rejuvenation to face what comes.

Sometimes when problems come too quickly to handle, I use a secret weapon. I am raised to a higher level by *not* resisting but turning it all over to the Holy Spirit. When this happens, worry and uncertainty are replaced with a new burst of confidence and energy. Then we—the Holy Spirit and I—take command of that particular day's problems.

Most of the time I can say with Paul, "I am troubled on every side but not crushed and broken. I am perplexed because I don't know why things happen as they do, but I don't give up and quit."

Other times I try to understand as Paul did when he heard the Lord say, "My grace is sufficient for you; for my strength is made perfect in weakness."

Epilog

THE PALE PONY REVISITED

Now I saw a pale horse,
and its rider's name was Death.
And there followed him another horse
whose rider's name was Hell.

The Pale Pony Created

The two mighty figures tossed fitfully upon the rough ground outside the smooth Garden walls. They stirred restlessly as the thin streaks of the New Dawn filtered over the unfamiliar horizon. Upon hearing the sound of diabolical laughter nearby, both awakened with a start.

First with wonder and then with amazement each examined his massive body and flexed his awesome muscles. Almost simultaneously each creature became aware of his own destructive power, and at the same time recognized similar punishing strength in the other. Each realized instinctively that he had a capacity for savage action to be directed against a foe which was common to them both.

Yet intuitively both knew that neither of them would choose the time and place to act. Strangely, they understood, too, that they had been created as allies, and that both were subservient to another angry, overriding force.

Suddenly their maker appeared before them. He called out,

"I am known by many names, but to you I will be called Lucifer!

"I have planned mighty deeds for you against the new blundering creature called Man.

"You," Lucifer announced to one figure, "shall be known as Death! You will be feared and avoided by Man. He will fight you with all his puny strength and cunning; yet you, Death, will always triumph at the end of Man's life. His lifetime will be like a vapor, but yours will never end. Because of your strength and authority some of them will call you the King of Darkness.

"I, the magnificent Lucifer, endow you with the power to Kill, to end every Man's life on what is known as Earth."

To the second figure Lucifer proclaimed, "You shall be called Hell! Many Men will fearfully refer to you as the Unseen State, quaking at your power against their permanent beings. Like Death, your life is eternal and your effects unknown to anyone but Lucifer. Men will tremble at your name!

"To some Men you will arrive before Death has his due. To all Men you will appear after Death has come. Time will not matter because you will always be ready to claim each Man's soul!

"I endow you, Hell, with the power to Chastise, Torment, and Punish—sometimes on the planet Earth and forever where you will abide with your subjects!

"Look now, Death and Hell, you have been given crushing powers against Man

> *to intimidate, to dismay,*
> *to frighten, to terrify,*
> *to frustrate, to afflict,*
> *to discourage, to overwhelm,*
> *to torture, to scourge,*
> *to crucify, to damn.*

"I myself will be near to direct you!

"From this very day until time ends," Lucifer continued, *"you have the gift of being where I want you to be at the precise moment that I have need of you. That power is available to both of you as part of my omnipotent plan.*

"See! At this very time I give you marvelous horses! They will whisk both of you across the face of Earth even to different places at the same instant of time.

"Death, yours is the mighty pale horse! Hell, the ghostly gray horse is yours to ride!

"There is even more, Mighty Servants! The great Lucifer gives you many helpers and strong weapons. Man, your foe, will call them demons, and they will be a regular part of your battle strategy when you wage war against Man for me. Meet and use these seven spirits: Loneliness, Frustration, Doubt, Fear, Pessimism, Despair, and Hopelessness!"

Then Lucifer shouted, *"Last, I show you my crowning stroke! A threat of your presence. A token of your coming visit. A harbinger of your impending victories!!*

"Death and Hell—see the masterpiece of torment which will work for you in ages to come! The foal of Death's pale horse and Hell's ghostly gray, the Pale Pony named Chronic Illness!!!"

And then Lucifer unleashed them all, leaving them alert and awaiting his call.

The Pale Pony Confronted

As if it were yesterday instead of over a decade ago, I remember the vicious predictions from the Pale Pony. As soon as it took recognizable form, it threatened,

You can no longer go where you want to go—whenever you care to—at the pace that you choose. I will be your constant companion. My name is Chronic Illness.

Fixing me with its unblinking, malevolent stare, it said,

The sentence of confinement, weakness, and pain is

not yours alone. Your wife and family, too, will suf-
fer, beginning slowly and then increasing to levels
that destroy! First you and then those who are close
to you.
Excitement and achievement? . . .
Never again will you have them like before!
It is useless to resist because defeat is all you can expect!

I thought about what the Pony had said, was afraid for me
and mine, and ran from him. I led Myra Sue and the boys
over every open trail, sought aid from those who claimed knowledge, and took cover when shelter was available—all to elude
the Pale Pony and its fearful predictions.

And yet the Pony stayed with us. Indeed it became increasingly clear that it had the power to weaken, to cripple, to
handicap. What's more, it shed a special kind of pain on Myra
Sue, so piercing that her own Pony trapped her. One day we
stopped running and looked squarely at our problems from
the Pony. I became excited about what it had revealed about
itself and its battle tactics.

As to the Pony—it was a witness of Evil in the World. As
long as I had known it, its words and actions reflected such
negative emotions as Envy, Jealousy of Joy, Malicious Oppres-
sion, Isolation, and Condemnation. Knowing the Pony's master
was the first step in meeting its attack.

Finding its source of power, however, certainly made the
Pony no less formidable or fear inspiring. It must have sensed
my awe at its demonstrated strength against Myra Sue and me
because the Pony began to boast:

"Since the beginning of time I have used the same
tactics to defeat Man and Woman! Surely it's evident
that I have succeeded in pushing more powerful people
than Ronald and Myra Sue Pruet off life's level table!"
Pausing for a malicious chuckle, it continued,
"I don't mind disclosing the very steps which will
destroy you both. After all, they have become polished
and proven through the ages!
"The first maneuver in prolonged illness is to bring

about separation. *Separation of man and wife from past joy, separation from past experience, separation from what's familiar!*

"The second deadly weapon is affliction. *Affliction with pain, affliction with weakness, affliction with loneliness!*

"The final crushing weapon is uncertainty about tomorrow. *Uncertainty about daily activity, uncertainty about money, uncertainty about life itself!*

"In every part of the battle, you will come to know and fear my allies. Some men call them demons; others dismiss them as emotions. No matter—we will divide your soul and body between us, and then turn you over to Death and Hell!

"I repeat, Defeat is all that you can expect!!"

Very quickly, we recognized that every aid we could find must be summoned for our all-out battles with unseen powers. We thought of everything we could *do,* since we had learned that there was no place to run and hide. We tried good deeds, sporadic prayers, heartfelt prayers, the wisdom of men, support from family and friends.

Through the years that have passed in our struggle with the Pale Pony and its allies, the tide of battle has surged and then ebbed. At times the complexion of the conflict has changed as delicately as the soft hues of a fading sunset—at others as quickly as the spirit of a summer rainstorm.

Often Myra Sue and I have been calm, strong, and victorious. Nevertheless, more times than we care to count, we have been distraught, weak, and defeated.

For the long fight, the sum of all that we can muster seems to be less than what the Pony brings to bear upon us.

Merciful Father, what can we do to overcome the boastful Pony's plan?

The Pale Pony Conquered

"Other than using every weapon that we can gather for our fight, what more can we do to win?" we asked desperately.

Then came the soothing answer, "Nothing else. It has already been done for you."

Then we remembered what Jesus said to His disciples just before He was crucified. He told them:

> *I am leaving you with a gift—peace of mind and heart. And the peace I give isn't fragile like the peace the world gives. So don't be troubled or afraid.*
>
> *I am the true Vine, and my Father is the Gardener. He lops off every branch that doesn't produce. And he prunes those branches that bear fruit for even larger crops. He has already tended you by pruning you back for greater strength and usefulness. . . ."*
>
> *Yes, I am the Vine, you are the branches. Whoever lives in Me and I in him shall produce a large crop of fruit. For apart from me you can't do a thing.*
>
> *I command that you love each other as much as I love you. And here is how to measure it—the greatest love is shown when a person lays down his life for his friends, and you are my friends if you obey me.*
>
> *You didn't choose me! I chose you! I appointed you to go and produce lovely fruit always, so that no matter what you ask from the Father, using my name, He will give it to you.*
>
> *Oh, there is so much more I want to tell you, but you can't understand it now. But when the Father sends the Comforter instead of me—and by the Comforter I mean the Holy Spirit—He will teach you much, as well as remind you of everything I myself have told you.*
>
> *In the world you will have many trials and sorrows, but cheer up, I have overcome the World!!*

Why, yes!! Centuries before He was crucified, the prophet Isaiah said of Jesus,

> *It was our grief He bore, our sorrows that weighed Him down. And we thought His troubles were a punishment from God for His own sins! But He was*

wounded and bruised for our sins. He was chastised
that we might have peace; He was lashed—and we
were healed!!

Myra Sue and I looked at each other in awe at the depth
of love and understanding that we found in His words. He
knows and cares about our struggles with Pale Ponies!

He *is* our Friend now and has been even *before* those foundations that Myra Sue told about were laid down!

Then we read more about what Jesus told His disciples after
His resurrection:

Death and Hell have no dominion over me!
I have destroyed the last enemy—Death!
I am alive for evermore and have the keys of Hell
and Death!
The devil sinned from the very beginning of time.
the reason that I came was to destroy the works of the
devil!!

Why, He was talking about Satan's whole arsenal against
Man! Those words are just as alive now as they were nearly
two thousand years ago!

Finally, John gave us the words that trumpeted Triumph:
"*Who is he that overcometh the World, but he that believeth*
that Jesus is the Son of God?"

At last we realized what He wanted us to know!

Our battles have already been won!!

We believe that Jesus conquered the Pale Pony when He
destroyed the works of the devil. He did it for those whom
He called to be His friends.